International Migration: Caring for Children and Families

Editors

STEPHEN LUDWIG
ANDREW P. STEENHOFF
JULIE M. LINTON

PEDIATRIC CLINICS
OF NORTH AMERICA

www.pediatric.theclinics.com

Consulting Editor
BONITA F. STANTON

June 2019 • Volume 66 • Number 3

ELSEVIER

1600 John F. Kennedy Boulevard ● Suite 1800 ● Philadelphia, Pennsylvania, 19103-2899

http://www.theclinics.com

THE PEDIATRIC CLINICS OF NORTH AMERICA Volume 66, Number 3
June 2019 ISSN 0031-3955, ISBN-13: 978-0-323-67868-1

Editor: Kerry Holland
Developmental Editor: Casey Potter

The Pediatric Clinics of North America (ISSN 0031-3955) is published bimonthly by Elsevier Inc., 360 Park Avenue South, New York, NY 10010-1710. Months of issue are February, April, June, August, October, and December. Periodicals postage paid at New York, NY and additional mailing offices. Subscription prices are $229.00 per year (US individuals), $653.00 per year (US institutions), $315.00 per year (Canadian individuals), $868.00 per year (Canadian institutions), $345.00 per year (international individuals), $868.00 per year (international institutions), $100.00 per year (US students and residents), and $165.00 per year (international and Canadian residents and students). To receive students/resident rare, orders must be accompanied by name of affiliated institution, date of term, and the signature of program/residency coordinator on institution letterhead. Orders will be billed at individual rate until proof of status is received. Foreign air speed delivery is included in all *Clinics* subscription prices. All prices are subject to change without notice. **POSTMASTER:** Send address changes to *The Pediatric Clinics of North America*, Elsevier Health Sciences Division, Subscription Customer Service, 3251 Riverport Lane, Maryland Heights, MO 63043. **Customer Service: 1-800-654-2452 (US and Canada). From outside of the US and Canada: 1-314-447-8871. Fax: 1-314-447-8029. For print support, E-mail: JournalsCustomerService-usa@elsevier.com. For online support, E-mail: JournalsOnlineSupport-usa@elsevier.com.**

Reprints. For copies of 100 or more, of articles in this publication, please contact the Commercial Reprints Department, Elsevier Inc., 360 Park Avenue South, New York, NY 10010-1710. Tel.: 212-633-3874; Fax: 212-633-3820; E-mail: reprints@elsevier.com.

The Pediatric Clinics of North America is also published in Spanish by McGraw-Hill Inter-americana Editores S.A., Mexico City, Mexico; in Portuguese by Riechmann and Affonso Editores, Rua Comandante Coelho 1085, CEP 21250, Rio de Janeiro, Brazil; and in Greek by Althayia SA, Athens, Greece.

The Pediatric Clinics of North America is covered in *MEDLINE/PubMed (Index Medicus), Excerpta Medica, Current Contents, Current Contents/Clinical Medicine, Science Citation Index, ASCA, ISI/BIOMED,* and *BIOSIS.*

Printed in the United States of America.

PROGRAM OBJECTIVE
The goal of the *Pediatric Clinics of North America* is to keep practicing physicians and residents up to date with current clinical practice in pediatrics by providing timely articles reviewing the state-of-the-art in patient care.

TARGET AUDIENCE
All practicing pediatricians, physicians and healthcare professionals who provide patient care to pediatric patients.

LEARNING OBJECTIVES
Upon completion of this activity, participants will be able to:
1. Review clinical tools for working both abroad and in the US with migrants
2. Discuss the history of immigration and the regulatory oversight of US immigration policies
3. Recognize communication barriers in refugee healthcare

ACCREDITATIONS
Physician Credit

The Elsevier Office of Continuing Medical Education (EOCME) is accredited by the Accreditation Council for Continuing Medical Education (ACCME) to provide continuing medical education for physicians.

The EOCME designates this enduring material for a maximum of 15 *AMA PRA Category 1 Credit*(s)™. Physicians should claim only the credit commensurate with the extent of their participation in the activity.

All other healthcare professionals requesting continuing education credit for this enduring material will be issued a certificate of participation.

ABP Maintenance of Certification Credit

Successful completion of this CME activity, which includes participation in the activity and individual assessment of and feedback to the learner, enables the learner to earn up to 15 MOC points in the American Board of Pediatrics' (ABP). Maintenance of Certification (MOC) program. It is the CME activity provider's responsibility to submit learner completion information to ACCME for the purpose of granting ABP MOC credit.

DISCLOSURE OF CONFLICTS OF INTEREST
The EOCME assesses conflict of interest with its instructors, faculty, planners, and other individuals who are in a position to control the content of CME activities. All relevant conflicts of interest that are identified are thoroughly vetted by EOCME for fair balance, scientific objectivity, and patient care recommendations. EOCME is committed to providing its learners with CME activities that promote improvements or quality in healthcare and not a specific proprietary business or a commercial interest.

The planning committee, staff, authors and editors listed below have identified no financial relationships or relationships to products or devices they or their spouse/life partner have with commercial interest related to the content of this CME activity:
Julia Burger, MD, MA; Martin Cetron, MD; Sarah K. Clarke, MSPH; Clare Clingain, BS; Adriana Deverlis, MPIA; Mary Fabio, MD, FAAP; Olanrewaju O. Falusi, MD; Ashleigh Hall, DO, MA; Kerry Holland; Anisa Ibrahim, MD; Janice Jaffe, PhD, CMI; Nora L. Jones, PhD; Alison Kemp; Julie M. Linton, MD, FAAP; Stephen Ludwig, MD, FAAP; Rajkumar Mayakrishnan; Ryan McAuley, MD, MPH; Tarissa Mitchell, MD; Raewyn Mutch, MBChB, DipRACOG, FRACP, PhD; Jennifer Nagda, JD; Lisa D. Parker, MSS; Drew L. Posey, MD, MPH; Sarah Poutasse, RN, FNP-BC; Kathleen A. Reeves, MD; Lauren Rogers-Sirin, PhD; Meera B. Siddharth, MD, FAAP; Esther Sin, MA; Selcuk R. Sirin, PhD; Andrew P. Steenhoff, MBBCh, DCH(UK), FCPaed(SA), FAAP; James A. Stockman III, MD; Chloe Turner, MD, FAAP; Michelle Weinberg, MD, MPH; Mary Brennan Wirshup, MD.

UNAPPROVED/OFF-LABEL USE DISCLOSURE
The EOCME requires CME faculty to disclose to the participants:
1. When products or procedures being discussed are off-label, unlabelled, experimental, and/or investigational (not US Food and Drug Administration [FDA] approved); and
2. Any limitations on the information presented, such as data that are preliminary or that represent ongoing research, interim analyses, and/or unsupported opinions. Faculty may discuss information about pharmaceutical agents that is outside of FDA-approved labelling. This information is intended solely for CME

and is not intended to promote off-label use of these medications. If you have any questions, contact the medical affairs department of the manufacturer for the most recent prescribing information.

TO ENROLL
To enroll in the *Pediatric Clinics of North America* Continuing Medical Education program, call customer service at 1-800-654-2452 or sign up online at http://www.theclinics.com/home/cme. The CME program is available to subscribers for an additional annual fee of USD 301.60.

METHOD OF PARTICIPATION
In order to claim credit, participants must complete the following:
1. Complete enrolment as indicated above.
2. Read the activity.
3. Complete the CME Test and Evaluation. Participants must achieve a score of 70% on the test. All CME Tests and Evaluations must be completed online.

In order to claim MOC points, participants must complete the following:
1. Complete steps listed above for claiming CME credit
2. Provide your specialty board ID#, birth date (MM/DD), and attestation.
3. Online MOC submission is only available for the American Board of pediatrics' (ABP) Maintenance of Certification (MOC) program

CME INQUIRIES/SPECIAL NEEDS
For all CME inquiries or special needs, please contact elsevierCME@elsevier.com

Contributors

CONSULTING EDITOR

BONITA F. STANTON, MD
Founding Dean, Hackensack Meridian School of Medicine at Seton Hall University, President, Academic Enterprise, Hackensack Meridian Health Robert C. and Laura C. Garrett Endowed Chair for the School of Medicine, Professor of Pediatrics, Nutley, New Jersey, USA

EDITORS

STEPHEN LUDWIG, MD, FAAP
Senior Director of Medical Education, Children's Hospital of Philadelphia, Professor of Pediatrics, Perelman School of Medicine, University of Pennsylvania, Philadelphia, Pennsylvania, USA

ANDREW P. STEENHOFF, MBBCh, DCH(UK), FCPaed(SA), FAAP
Medical Director of Global Health, Children's Hospital of Philadelphia, Assistant Professor of Pediatrics, Perelman School of Medicine, University of Pennsylvania, Philadelphia, Pennsylvania, USA

JULIE M. LINTON, MD, FAAP
Clinical Associate Professor, University of South Carolina School of Medicine Greenville, Prisma Health Upstate Children's Hospital, Greenville, South Carolina, USA; Adjunct Faculty, Wake Forest School of Medicine, Winston-Salem, North Carolina, USA

AUTHORS

JULIA BURGER, MD, MA
Department of Pediatrics, Lewis Katz School of Medicine at Temple University, Philadelphia, Pennsylvania, USA

MARTIN CETRON, MD
Director, Division of Global Migration and Quarantine, Centers for Disease Control and Prevention, Georgia, USA

SARAH K. CLARKE, MSPH
Coordinator, Society of Refugee Healthcare Providers, Calgary, Alberta, Canada

CLARE CLINGAIN, BS
Master's Candidate, Department of Applied Statistics, Social Science, and Humanities, Steinhardt School of Culture, Education, and Human Development, New York University, New York, New York, USA

ADRIANA DEVERLIS, MPIA
Global Health Center, Children's Hospital of Philadelphia, Philadelphia, Pennsylvania, USA

MARY FABIO, MD, FAAP
Clinical Assistant Professor of Pediatrics, Perelman School of Medicine, University of Pennsylvania, Attending Physician, Children's Hospital of Philadelphia, Karabots Pediatric Care Center, Philadelphia, Pennsylvania, USA

OLANREWAJU O. FALUSI, MD
Assistant Professor of Pediatrics, The George Washington University School of Medicine and Health Sciences, Children's National Health System, Washington, DC, USA

ASHLEIGH HALL, DO, MA
Department of Pediatrics, Lewis Katz School of Medicine at Temple University, Philadelphia, Pennsylvania, USA

ANISA IBRAHIM, MD
Clinical Assistant Professor, Department of Pediatrics, University of Washington, Harborview Medical Center, Seattle, Washington, USA

JANICE JAFFE, PhD, CMI
Medical Interpreter, Maine Medical Center, Visiting Associate Professor, Hispanic Studies, Department of Romance Languages and Literatures, Bowdoin College, Brunswick, Maine, USA

NORA L. JONES, PhD
Center for Bioethics, Urban Health, and Policy, Lewis Katz School of Medicine at Temple University, Philadelphia, Pennsylvania, USA

JULIE M. LINTON, MD, FAAP
Clinical Associate Professor, University of South Carolina School of Medicine Greenville, Prisma Health Upstate Children's Hospital, Greenville, South Carolina, USA; Adjunct Faculty, Wake Forest School of Medicine, Winston-Salem, North Carolina, USA

STEPHEN LUDWIG, MD, FAAP
Senior Director of Medical Education, Children's Hospital of Philadelphia, Professor of Pediatrics, Perelman School of Medicine, University of Pennsylvania, Philadelphia, Pennsylvania, USA

RYAN McAULEY, MD, MPH
Instructor, Division of Hematology/Oncology, Department of Medicine, Perelman School of Medicine, University of Pennsylvania, Philadelphia, Pennsylvania, USA

TARISSA MITCHELL, MD
Medical Officer, Immigrant, Refugee, and Migrant Health Branch, Division of Global Migration and Quarantine, Centers for Disease Control and Prevention, Atlanta, Georgia, USA

RAEWYN MUTCH, MBChB, DipRACOG, FRACP, PhD
Consultant Paediatrician, Refugee Health and General Paediatrics, Department of General Paediatrics, Perth Children's Hospital, Clinical Associate Professor, School of Medicine, Dentistry and Health Sciences, University of Western Australia, Perth, Western Australia, Australia

JENNIFER NAGDA, JD
Policy Director, Young Center for Immigrant Children's Rights, Chicago, Illinois, USA

LISA D. PARKER, MSS
Founder, Peace Day Philly and United Nations Representative, Peace Day Philly, Philadelphia, Pennsylvania, USA

DREW L. POSEY, MD, MPH
Medical Officer, Immigrant, Refugee, and Migrant Health Branch, Division of Global Migration and Quarantine, Centers for Disease Control and Prevention, Atlanta, Georgia, USA

SARAH POUTASSE, RN, FNP-BC
Community Volunteers in Medicine, West Chester, Pennsylvania, USA

KATHLEEN A. REEVES, MD
Center for Bioethics, Urban Health, and Policy, Lewis Katz School of Medicine at Temple University, Philadelphia, Pennsylvania, USA

LAUREN ROGERS-SIRIN, PhD
Associate Professor, Department of Psychology, College of Staten Island, The City University of New York, Staten Island, New York, USA

MEERA B. SIDDHARTH, MD, FAAP
Clinical Assistant Professor of Pediatrics, Department of Emergency Medicine, Perelman School of Medicine, University of Pennsylvania, Urgent Care Attending, Children's Hospital of Philadelphia, Philadelphia, Pennsylvania, USA

ESTHER SIN, MA
Doctoral Candidate, Department of Applied Psychology, Steinhardt School of Culture, Education, and Human Development, New York University, New York, New York, USA

SELCUK R. SIRIN, PhD
Professor, Department of Applied Psychology, Steinhardt School of Culture, Education, and Human Development, New York University, New York, New York, USA

ANDREW P. STEENHOFF, MBBCh, DCH(UK), FCPaed(SA), FAAP
Medical Director of Global Health, Children's Hospital of Philadelphia, Assistant Professor of Pediatrics, Perelman School of Medicine, University of Pennsylvania, Philadelphia, Pennsylvania, USA

JAMES A. STOCKMAN III, MD
Consultant, American Board of Pediatrics, Chapel Hill, North Carolina, USA

CHLOE TURNER, MD, FAAP
Medical Director of Pediatrics, Unity Health Care, Inc., Washington, DC, USA; Clinical Assistant Professor, A.T. Still University of Health Sciences, Mesa, Arizona, USA

MICHELLE WEINBERG, MD, MPH
Senior Medical Officer, Immigrant, Refugee, and Migrant Health Branch, Division of Global Migration and Quarantine, Centers for Disease Control and Prevention, Atlanta, Georgia, USA

MARY BRENNAN WIRSHUP, MD, FAAFP
Community Volunteers in Medicine, West Chester, Pennsylvania, USA

Contents

This article briefly covers the history of immigration from the US perspective, including the demographic variation over time and the ever-changing policies. Displaced children and their families are facing increasing challenges to their health and overall wellbeing. Since enactment of the Immigration and Nationality Act of 1965, the needs of minors have been caught up in complex immigration policy. Recognition of the unique needs of minors and the Dreamers must be addressed as part of comprehensive immigration reform or in more targeted legislative proposals. The challenges posed by the magnitude and scope of the immigration problem are discussed.

This article briefly examines the scope of international migration–related issues and issues related to the migration of individuals and families across the southern border of the United States. Immigration issues include designing oversight policies consistent with international treaties yet tailored to suit the unique circumstances of recipient countries; integrating refugees and asylum seekers; and dealing with undocumented foreigners who have gained entry across a border. Most importantly, ways must be found that allow accompanied and unaccompanied minors to live a full and healthy existence as they wend their way through a most difficult time in their lives.

Migration and forced displacement are at record levels in today's geopolitical environment; ensuring the health of migrating populations and the health security of asylum and receiving countries is critically important. Overseas screening, treatment, and vaccination during planned migration to the United States represents one successful model. These strategies have improved tuberculosis detection and treatment, reducing rates in the United States; decreased transmission and importation of vaccine-preventable diseases; prevented morbidity and mortality from parasitic diseases among refugees; and saved health costs. We describe the work of CDC's Division of Global Migration and Quarantine and partners in developing and implementing these strategies.

clinical care and offer clinical tools to achieve the provision of accessible, comprehensive, high-quality care within a family-centered medical home.

Immigration laws and policies, as well as related media and public discourse, have a direct and significant effect on the health and well-being of children and families. The purpose of this article is to identify the impact of family immigration status and immigration laws on children's health, to understand the legal system that immigrant children face, and to describe opportunities for health care professionals to engage in advocacy at the systems level, from the local community to Capitol Hill.

In this article, the authors provide an overview of the current global and US debates on immigration as a key developmental context for immigrant-origin youth. Relying on a conceptual framework that highlights both risk and protective factors, the authors provide evidence from their longitudinal study that empirically links acculturative stress to key mental health outcomes during adolescence. They conclude with a discussion of clinical implications of their work with an emphasis on what is needed to meet the growing mental health needs of immigrant youth.

This article focuses on the resiliency of refugee families and the various ways that pediatric practitioners can use and strengthen those resiliencies in the course of pediatric health care delivery. It reviews common stressors experienced by refugees, information about the concept of resilience, aspects of culturally responsive health care, and clinical recommendations. In addition, 3 cases are presented that highlight both resiliencies of refugee families and successful interventions by pediatric health care providers within the pediatric refugee clinic at the Children's Hospital of Philadelphia.

Research demonstrates that language and cultural barriers negatively affect care for patients with limited English proficiency, resulting in significant and costly health disparities. Legal standards emphasize working with qualified interpreters, but training for providers on communicating effectively through interpreters is inconsistent. Knowing the difference between a translator and interpreter, an interpreter's role, and who can be a qualified interpreter are key for providers. Generally accepted best practice for working with medical interpreters includes tips for before, during, and after an interpreted encounter. Potential solutions exist for ethical dilemmas and challenges commonly experienced when working with interpreters.

Globally, significant progress in health equity for children has been made, but much work remains. This article discusses why and how the pediatric community in North America is building a global health (GH) workforce, for domestic "local global" and "international global child health" settings. With a focus on children and families, training this workforce entails attaining GH competencies in medical students, residents, fellows, allied medical professionals, and upskilling current practitioners. The authors highlight currently available training approaches and resources for each group. Global child health is now within the purview of every pediatrician in North America.

PEDIATRIC CLINICS OF NORTH AMERICA

FORTHCOMING ISSUES

August 2019
Hospital Medicine and Clinical Education
Nancy Spector and Amy Starmer, *Editors*

October 2019
Pediatric Orthopedics
Paul T. Haynes, *Editor*

December 2019
Substance Abuse
David R. Rosenberg and Leslie H. Lundahl, *Editors*

RECENT ISSUES

April 2018
Current Advances in Neonatal Care
Beena G. Sood and Dara D. Brodsky, *Editors*

February 2019
Clinical Disorders of the Kidney
James C. Chan, *Editor*

December 2018
Pediatric Emergency Medicine
Prashant Mahajan, *Editor*

SERIES OF RELATED INTEREST

Clinics in Perinatology
https://www.perinatology.theclinics.com/

THE CLINICS ARE AVAILABLE ONLINE!
Access your subscription at:
www.theclinics.com

PEDIATRIC CLINICS OF
NORTH AMERICA

Foreword

Delivering on the Promise of the Statue of Liberty

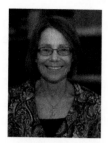

Bonita F. Stanton, MD
Consulting Editor

America is a nation that prides itself on its multinational origins, a pride that is reflected in iconic figures, such as the Statue of Liberty. A large percentage of our pediatric workforce is committed to serving children in need, wherever they may be. The call for humanitarian care can arise in the home countries of vulnerable or persecuted populations (or the neighboring countries to which the families are fleeing), countries ravaged by international war or internal conflict, famine, natural disasters, chronic poverty, or acutely failing economies, or a mixture of the above. In each of these cases, pediatric health care providers will travel abroad, whether with established relief and/or humanitarian groups, with sponsorship from religious groups or other organizations committed to humanity (such as the Red Cross, Doctors without Borders, to mention but a few), or on their own initiative. As importantly, the need for such care within the borders of our own country is equally compelling. In fact, perhaps even *more* compelling, given the significant numbers of young children accompanying their families seeking refuge in the United States has been increasing in recent years.[1,2]

Reflecting commitment to supporting their workforce in its efforts to optimize the care provided, many departments of pediatrics, pediatric professional agencies (including the American Academy of Pediatrics, the American Board of Pediatrics, and numerous pediatric specialty boards), have developed platforms for effective practices in settings around the globe. These platforms are designed to prepare the practitioners to effectively react to the needs of children in stressed conditions. Supporting these platforms are an increasing number of needed guidelines, curricula, textbooks, educational meetings, special programs, and training opportunities designed to facilitate effective care in unfamiliar settings.

To date, much of the emphasis has been on providing the materials to support US pediatric providers traveling abroad. However, the needs at home to adequately address immigrant children are equally compelling. Supporting the rapidly growing

Pediatr Clin N Am 66 (2019) xv–xvi
https://doi.org/10.1016/j.pcl.2019.03.016
0031-3955/19/© 2019 Published by Elsevier Inc.

needs and interest among pediatric practitioners responding to the needs of migrant children who have found their way to the United States, the current volume of *Pediatric Clinics of North America* addresses the children's many medical, social, community, economic, psychosocial, and legal issues. The authors are experienced in addressing this vast array of issues and knowledgeable with regard to optimizing outcomes. The seventeen articles comprising this issue will enable all pediatricians in the United States to adequately address these issues with competence among the growing number of refugee children in pediatric practices across the United States.

Bonita F. Stanton, MD
Hackensack Meridian School of Medicine
at Seton Hall University
340 Kingsland Street, Building 123
Nutley, NJ 07110, USA

E-mail address:
bonita.stanton@shu.edu

REFERENCES

1. Migration Policy Institute. Rising child migration to the USA. Available at: https://www.migrationpolicy.org/programs/us-immigration-policy-program/rising-child-migration-united-states. Accessed March 15, 2019.
2. Zong J, Batalova J, Burrow M, et al. Frequently requested statistics on immigrants and immigration in the United States. Migration information source: spotlight, March 14, 2019. Migration Policy Institute. Available at: https://www.migrationpolicy.org/article/frequently-requested-statistics-immigrants-and-immigration-united-states. Accessed March 15, 2019.

Preface

Immigrant and Refugee Health: Why this Topic? Why now?

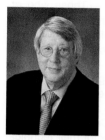
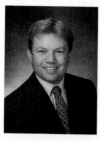
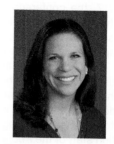

Stephen Ludwig, MD, FAAP

Andrew P. Steenhoff, MBBCh, DCH(UK), FCPaed(SA), FAAP

Julie M. Linton, MD, FAAP

Editors

CHOP

Each year the Global Health Department of the Children's Hospital of Philadelphia plans a Global Health Conference for health care professionals. Each year we try to select an important and relevant topic for the meeting. In 2016, we began the planning for the 2017 conference. In our multidisciplinary planning group, the decision was unanimous. We selected "Immigrant and Refugee Health" as our theme. We did this for several reasons. The topic seemed to be both current and even urgent. Current because of significant changes our government was making relevant to immigration policy. Current because millions of immigrants without legal status were criminalized and faced threatened deportation; Deferred Action for Childhood Arrivals youth were placed in limbo, and the refugee resettlement program was vastly reduced. Families faced a climate of fear and uncertainty, reluctant to seek health care services or presenting with physical and psychological signs reflective of stress. Only the most serious of childhood illnesses would come to our attention. The situation was urgent, as never before in history had there been so many displaced persons around the world. Some estimated 50 million displaced children, and 28 million of those were displaced by conflict. Children represented 50% of all refugees.

Global Health is about health equity: health not only of those beyond our borders but also within our communities. As a sanctuary city, Philadelphia was the home to many of these children, and our community was trying to provide the best health care possible. Our hospital was well integrated in this effort. Our outpatient centers were providing care for children who had been born in other countries and preferred languages that were new to us. Some of our trainees were doing volunteer work in community-based clinics. Others were electing to take part in global health electives around the world. Julio Frenk and colleagues[1] wrote,

> Global Health should not be viewed as foreign health, but rather as the health of the global population. Global Health should be understood not as a manifestation of dependence, but rather as the product of interdependence.

In October 2017, the conference was held for 200 attendees. Those who attended heard thought-provoking lectures, participated in workshops, engaged with poster presenters, and had a chance to network with colleagues. With the conference completed, we sought a way to expand our impact and share what we had gained. Thus, the idea of this issue emerged. Many of our speakers and presenters readily agreed to put their presentations into writing, and the articles that appear in this issue are evidence of their commitment. As editors, we deeply thank them for doing the important work not once but twice. We also wish to thank Dr Bonnie Stanton for her encouragement of the project and Casey Marie Potter and the production staff of the *Pediatric Clinics of North America* for their technical support and advice.

The Global Health Task Force of the American Board of Pediatrics has proposed the following:

> The health of children across the world is critical to the continued and improved existence of our world as we know it. Therefore, this outcome is in part the responsibility of all pediatricians and of every department of pediatrics and pediatric governing body.

We hope that our conference and this publication are small steps in meeting that responsibility.

Stephen Ludwig, MD, FAAP
Children's Hospital of Philadelphia
Perelman School of Medicine
University of Pennsylvania
3401 Civic Center Boulevard
Philadelphia, PA 19104, USA

Andrew P. Steenhoff, MBBCh, DCH(UK),
FCPaed(SA), FAAP
Children's Hospital of Philadelphia
Perelman School of Medicine
University of Pennsylvania
3401 Civic Center Boulevard
Philadelphia, PA 19104, USA

Julie M. Linton, MD, FAAP
University of South Carolina School of Medicine Greenville
Prisma Health Upstate Children's Hospital
Wake Forest School of Medicine
1200 North Martin Luther King Jr Drive
Winston-Salem, NC 27101, USA

E-mail addresses:
ludwig@email.chop.edu (S. Ludwig)
steenhoff@email.chop.edu (A.P. Steenhoff)
Julie.linton@prismahealth.org (J.M. Linton)

REFERENCE

1. Frenk J, Gomez-Dantes O, Moon S. From sovereignty to solidarity: a renewed concept of global health for an era of complex interdependence. Lancet 2014; 383:94–7.

Coming to America: Regulatory Oversight of United States Immigration Policies: A Brief History

James A. Stockman III, MD

KEYWORDS

- Immigration • Slavery • Migrants • Refugees
- Immigration and Nationality Act of 1965
- Immigration Reform and Control Act of 1986 • DACA

KEY POINTS

- Relief immigration services in recipient countries have been stretched to their limits, particularly when it comes to displaced children, many of whom travel unaccompanied and who face immigration policies that are not in their best interest.
- Between 500,000 to 650,000 Africans were brought to America and sold into slavery between the seventeenth and nineteenth centuries.
- A major wave of immigration occurred from 1815 to 1865. Most of these newcomers hailed from Northern and Western Europe. Approximately one-third came from Ireland, which experienced a massive famine in the mid-nineteenth century.
- Between 1880 and 1920, a time of rapid industrialization and urbanization, America received more than 20 million immigrants.
- In 1917, the US Congress enacted the first widely restrictive immigration law.

INTRODUCTION

Turmoil throughout many parts of the world has launched 1 of the longest periods of resettlements in the history of mankind. Relief immigration services in recipient countries have been stretched to their limits, particularly when it comes to displaced children, many of whom travel unaccompanied and who face immigration policies that are not in their best interest. This article briefly covers the history of immigration from the perspective of the United States, including the marked variation over time in those entering the country and our nation's changing immigration policies, up to the current time, a time in which displaced children and their families from Mexico, Central

---

Disclosure Statement: The author has nothing to disclose.
American Board of Pediatrics, 111 Silver Cedar Court, Chapel Hill, NC 27514, USA
E-mail address: jstockman@abpeds.org

America, the Middle East, and elsewhere are facing increasing challenges to their health and overall wellbeing as they navigate their way to our borders. The unique challenges posed by the sheer magnitude and scope of the immigration problem are discussed.

HISTORY OF MIGRATION TO NORTH AMERICA

Ours is indeed a nation of immigrants, starting with the first inhabitants who likely crossed the land bridge from Asia to North America. The first settlement of the Americas most likely began when Paleolithic hunter-gatherers entered North America from the North Asian Mammoth steppe via the Beringia land bridge, which had formed between (**Fig. 1**).[1,2] The earliest populations in the Americas, before roughly 10,000 years ago, are known as Paleo-Indians, the ancestors of the current Native American population and the Indian populations of Central and South America.

Millennia later, by the 1500s AD, the first Europeans, led by the Spanish and French, had begun establishing settlements in what would become the United States. The reasons for the subsequent migration to North America were many and principally included freedom to practice one's faith; economic opportunities; flight from violence elsewhere in the world; and, for many, indentured servitude, including slavery. In 1607, the English founded their first permanent settlement in present-day America at Jamestown in the Virginia Colony. In 1620, roughly 100 people, later known as the Pilgrims fled religious persecution in Europe and arrived at present-day Plymouth, Massachusetts, where they established a colony. They were soon followed by a larger group seeking religious freedom, the Puritans, who established the Massachusetts Bay Colony. By some estimates, 20,000 Puritans migrated to the region in the seventeenth century.[3]

In the 1700s, a larger share of immigrants came to America seeking economic opportunities. However, because the price of passage was steep, an estimated one-half or more of the white Europeans who made the voyage did so by becoming indentured servants. Although some people voluntarily indentured themselves, others were kidnapped in European cities and forced into servitude in America. Additionally, thousands of English convicts were shipped across the Atlantic as indentured servants. A group of immigrants who arrived against their will during the colonial period were black slaves from West Africa. The earliest records of slavery in America include a group of approximately 20 Africans who were forced into indentured servitude in Jamestown, Virginia, in 1619. By 1680, there were some 7000 African slaves in the American colonies, a number that ballooned to 700,000 by 1790, according to some estimates. Although the exact numbers will never be known, it is believed that between 500,000 to 650,000 Africans were brought to America and sold into slavery between the seventeenth and nineteenth centuries. The end of the Civil War in 1865 resulted in the emancipation of approximately 4 million slaves.[4]

A major wave of immigration occurred from 1815 to 1865. Most of these newcomers hailed from Northern and Western Europe. Approximately one-third came from Ireland, which experienced a massive famine in the mid-nineteenth century. In the 1840s, almost half of America's immigrants were from Ireland alone. Between 1820 and 1930, some 4.5 million Irish migrated to the United States. Typically impoverished, these Irish immigrants settled near their point of arrival in cities along the East Coast. Also, in the nineteenth century, the United States received some 5 million German immigrants. Many of them journeyed to the present-day Midwest to buy farms or congregate in cities such as Milwaukee, St. Louis, and Cincinnati. In the national census of 2000, more Americans claimed German ancestry than any other group.

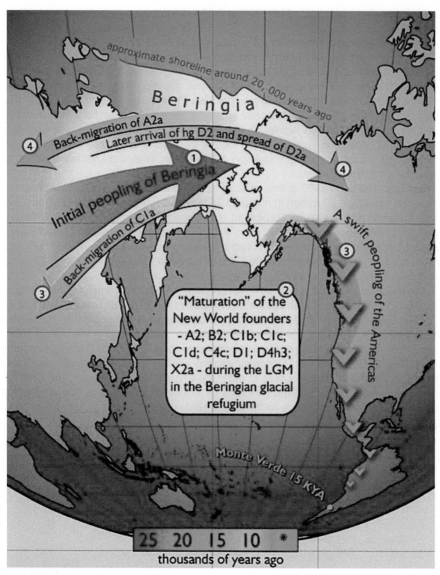

Fig. 1. Maternal gene-flow in and out of Beringia. (*From* Tamm E, Kivisild T, Reidla M, et al. Beringian standstill and spread of native American founders. PLoS One 2007;2(9):e829.)

The large influx of immigrants into the United States in the 1800s resulted in anti-immigrant sentiment among certain factions of America's native-born. New arrivals were often seen as unwanted competition for jobs. Many Catholics, especially the Irish, experienced discrimination for their religious beliefs. In the 1850s, the anti-immigrant, anti-Catholic American Party (also called the Know-Nothings) tried to severely curb immigration and even ran a candidate, former US President Millard Fillmore (1800–1874), in the presidential election of 1856. To many nativists the Catholic Church presented tyranny and allegiance to another authority (the Pope). As immigration from Ireland continued, nativist groups formed in many large cities. Anti-Irish riots broke out in Philadelphia in 1944 resulting in 15 to 20 deaths and the burning of a Catholic Church.[5]

Prejudice against other immigrant groups was also seen in the mid-nineteenth century. Chinese immigrants first flocked to the United States in the 1850s, eager to escape the economic chaos in China and to try their luck at the California gold rush. Chinese laborers were employed in the commercial mining of gold. When the Gold Rush ended, Chinese Americans were considered cheap labor. Some 25,000 Chinese had migrated to California by the early 1850s.[6] One of the very first significant restrictive pieces of immigration legislation at the Federal level was the Chinese Exclusion Act of 1882, which banned Chinese laborers from coming to America. Californians had agitated for the new law, blaming the Chinese, who were willing to work for less, for a decline in wages.[7]

Between 1880 and 1920, a time of rapid industrialization and urbanization, America received more than 20 million immigrants. In the 1890s, most arrivals were from Central, Eastern, and Southern Europe. In that decade alone, some 600,000 Italians migrated to America, and by 1920 more than 4 million had entered the United States. Jews from Eastern Europe fleeing religious persecution also arrived in large numbers; more than 2 million entered the United States between 1880 and 1920. In 1907 alone, approximately 1.3 million people entered the country legally.

The outbreak of World War I (1914–1918) caused a decline in immigration. Immigration also plummeted during the global depression of the 1930s and during World War II (1939–1945). Between 1930 and 1950, America's foreign-born population decreased from 14.2 to 10.3 million. The lowest percentage of foreign born in the United States population in the last 100 years was observed in the US Census Bureau records of 1970 (**Fig. 2**). After the war, Congress passed special legislation enabling refugees from Europe and the Soviet Union to enter the United States. Following the Communist revolution in Cuba in 1959, hundreds of thousands of refugees from that island nation also gained admittance to the United States.

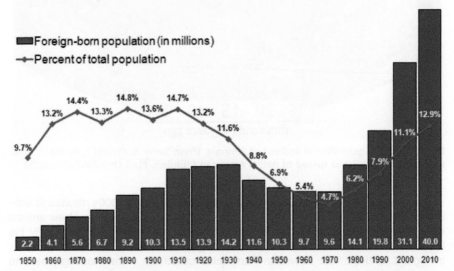

Fig. 2. Foreign-born population and percentage of total population for the United States: 1850 to 2010. (*From* US Census Bureau, Census of Population, 1850 to 2000, and the American Community Survey, 2010. Available at: https://www.census.gov/newsroom/pdf/cspan_fb_slides.pdf. Accessed March 20, 2019.)

When Congress passed the Immigration and Nationality Act (INA) in 1965, which did away with quotas based on nationality and allowed Americans to sponsor relatives from their countries of origin, the nation experienced a major shift in immigration patterns. Today, many US immigrants come from Asia and Latin America rather than Europe. Since the passage of the INA of 1965, the foreign-born population of the United States has increased 4-fold to 43.7 million in 2016 with a corresponding increase in the percentage of immigrants in the country's overall population (**Fig. 3**). About 1 in 4 children younger than 18 years old in the United States have at least 1 foreign-born parent. The trends toward immigration from individuals and families from south of the US border continues, now in part driven by refugee migration from Central America.

PAST AND CURRENT IMMIGRATION POLICIES: THEIR IMPACT ON IMMIGRANTS ENTERING THE UNITED STATES
Early Immigration Laws: Eighteenth and Nineteenth Centuries

America generally encouraged relatively free and open immigration during the eighteenth and the early part of the nineteenth centuries, not formulating lasting immigration policies until the late 1800s. Until then, there was relatively little in the way of federal legislative oversight of entry into the United States from foreign countries. What little legislation there was tended to impose limits that favored Europeans. A 1790 law was the first to specify who could become a citizen. This was the US Naturalization Law, passed on March 6, 1790.[8] The law limited naturalization to immigrants who were free white persons of good character. It thus excluded American Indians, indentured servants, slaves, free blacks, and (later) Asians, although free blacks were allowed citizenship at the state level in certain states. Immigrants had to have lived in the United States for at least 2 years before becoming eligible for citizenship. The Emancipation Proclamation freed all blacks but actual citizenship was not extended to those of African origin until 1870. After several states passed their own

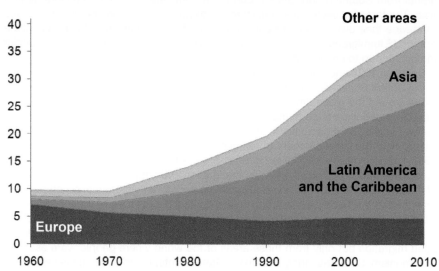

Fig. 3. Foreign-born population by region of birth: 1960 to 2010 (numbers in millions). Note: Other areas includes Africa, Northern America, Oceania, born at sea, and not reported. (*From* US Census Bureau, Census of Population, 1850 to 2000, and the American Community Survey, 2010. Available at: https://www.census.gov/newsroom/pdf/cspan_fb_slides.pdf. Accessed March 20, 2019.)

immigration laws following the Civil War, the Supreme Court in 1875 declared regulation of immigration a federal responsibility.

Starting in 1875, a series of restrictions on immigration were enacted. They included bans on criminals, people with contagious diseases, polygamists, anarchists, beggars, and importers of prostitutes. The Chinese Exclusion Act of 1882 and Alien Contract Labor laws of 1885 and 1887 prohibited certain laborers from immigrating to the United States.[9] The general Immigration Act of 1882 levied a head tax of 50 cents on each immigrant and blocked (or excluded) the entry of idiots, lunatics, convicts, and persons likely to become a public charge.[10]

Later Immigration Laws: Twentieth and Twenty-First Centuries

In 1917, the US Congress enacted the first widely restrictive immigration law.[11] The uncertainty generated over national security during World War I made it possible for Congress to pass this legislation. It included several important provisions that paved the way for the later Immigration Act of 1924. The Immigration Act of 1917 (also known as the Asiatic Barred Zone Act) implemented a restrictive literacy test that required immigrants older than 16 years old to demonstrate basic reading comprehension in any language (**Fig. 4**). It also increased the tax paid by new immigrants on arrival and allowed immigration officials to exercise more discretion in making decisions about whom to exclude. Finally, the Act excluded from entry anyone born in a geographically defined Asiatic Barred Zone except for Japanese and Filipinos.

The Immigration Act of 1924 (the Johnson Reed Act) was a landmark piece of immigration legislation signed into law by President Coolidge that limited the number of immigrants allowed entry into the United States through a national origins quota.[12] The quota provided immigration visas to 2% of the total number of people of each nationality in the United States as of the 1890 national census. The Act unequivocally favored immigrants from Western Europe. The Act also swung the doors closed to most immigrants from Southern and Eastern Europe. It completely excluded immigrants from Asia. The target of exclusions was intended to be the poor workers who were trying to escape their own society for economic opportunity. Years later, following calls to reform US immigration policy, the INA of 1965 finally ended the quota system, opening the country up to immigrants of other nations.

Between 1924 and 1965, there were other significant changes in immigration rates in the United States. During the Second World War, it was very difficult for people to move around the globe. Immigration almost came to a standstill. In the aftermath of the War, there were large numbers of refugees and displaced persons as a result of the war and Nazi persecution. In 1948, Congress passed a refugee relief bill that did little to help the large numbers of refugees attempting to settle in North America. In 1952, legislation allowed a limited number of visas for most Asian nationals. Congress recodified and combined all previous immigration and naturalization laws into the INA of 1952.[13] The 1952 law removed all racial barriers to immigration and naturalization and granted the same preference to husbands as it did to wives of American citizens. However, the INA retained the national origins quotas.

By the 1950s, migration was also a Cold War issue, and the United States encouraged migration but only from those areas of the world where people were escaping Communism. Other than that, The United States continued to observe the restrictions of the Reed-Johnson Act. There were 2 Cold War exceptions. One was in 1956 because of the Hungarian uprising, then again in 1959 because of Fidel Castro's ascent in Cuba.

It was very clear to some policymakers, including John F. Kennedy, who was pushing for reform at the time of his assassination, that the American immigration policies

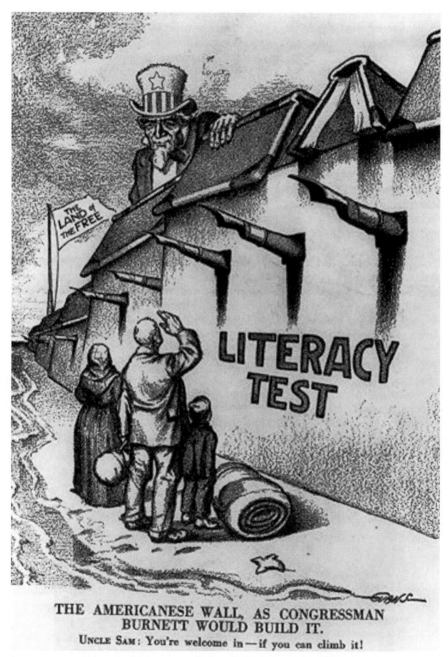

THE AMERICANESE WALL, AS CONGRESSMAN
BURNETT WOULD BUILD IT.

UNCLE SAM: You're welcome in — if you can climb it!

Fig. 4. A cartoonist's interpretation of the Immigration Act of 1917. (*From* Library of Congress. Available at: https://www.loc.gov/resource/cph.3b00563/. Accessed March 20, 2019.)

were too restrictive and unjust. In 1965 a combination of political, social, and geopolitical factors led to the passage of the landmark INA of 1965, signed by President Johnson. This act created a new system favoring family reunification and skilled immigrants, rather than country quotas[14] (**Fig. 5**).

This major change in US quota policy greatly altered the ethnic makeup of immigrants entering the United States during the late twentieth and early twenty-first centuries, and prompted a massive increase in total immigration. The law did impose the first limits on immigration from the Western Hemisphere. Before then, Latin Americans had been allowed to enter the United States without many restrictions. Since enactment of the INA of 1965, immigration has been dominated by people born in Asia and Latin America, rather than Europe. The INA of 1965 eliminated hard quotas on countries previously considered undesirable and ushered in a new era of ethnic, racial, and religious diversity. Although, in its first iteration, the law privileged skilled and educated workers, in its final iteration, it was biased toward family unification. The children, spouses, and siblings of legal residents took precedence, along with scientists, artists, professionals, and skilled manual workers. In the first years of its enactment, the new law opened the door to large numbers of professionals, particularly from Asia and the Asia-Pacific region. Whereas fewer than 2% of immigrants in 1900 qualified as skilled workers, by 1973 roughly 10% met that qualification. More than 50,000 physicians and nurses immigrated to the United States between 1969 and 1973 alone, most of them from countries such as the Philippines, South Korea, Pakistan, and China. Within 2 decades, upward of 80% of staff physicians at some New York hospitals were Asian immigrants. The same pattern was on display in other professions, particularly in the science, technology, engineering, and mathematics (STEM) fields.

The 1965 law's emphasis on family unification meant that large numbers of unskilled workers benefited as well, including many siblings and parents of skilled professionals. Of Chinese residents who arrived in the United States before 1970, fewer than 3% lived below the poverty line in their home country. Of those who came after 1975, roughly one-quarter had been poor.

Several laws since 1965 have focused on refugees, paving the way for the entrance of Indochinese refugees fleeing war violence in the 1970s. Later, there came relief for other nationalities, including Chinese, Nicaraguans, and Haitians. A 1990 law created the temporary protective status that has shielded immigrants, mainly Central Americans, from deportation to countries facing natural disasters, armed conflicts, or other extraordinary conditions.

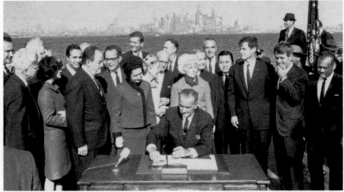

President Lyndon B. Johnson signing the Immigration and Nationality Act of 1965, which substantially changed U.S. immigration policy toward non-Europeans. Johnson made a point of signing the legislation near the base of the Statue of Liberty, which had long stood as a symbol of welcome to immigrants. Lower Manhattan can be seen in the background. *(Lyndon B. Johnson Library Collection/Yoichi R. Okamoto)*

Fig. 5. President Lyndon Johnson signing the INA of 1965. (*Courtesy of* Yoichi Okamoto, Lyndon B. Johnson Library.)

In 1986, Congress enacted another major law, the Immigration Reform and Control Act, which granted legalization to millions of unauthorized immigrants, mainly from Latin America, who met certain conditions (**Fig. 6**).[15] The law also imposed sanctions on employers who hired unauthorized immigrants. Subsequent laws in 1996, 2002, and 2006 were responses to concerns about terrorism and unauthorized immigration. These measures emphasized border control, prioritized enforcement of laws on hiring immigrants, and tightened admissions eligibility.

Lawmakers had been trying to get the Development, Relief, and Education for Alien Minors (DREAM) Act passed since at least 2001 with no success. In June 2012, using the power of Executive Action, President Barack Obama launched the Deferred Action for Childhood Arrivals (DACA) program to provide reprieve from deportation to young people who came to the United States as children.[16] The DACA program was a temporary measure until more comprehensive immigration reform for minors could be enacted. When the DACA program was put into place, individuals who arrived in the country before their sixteenth birthday were eligible for the DACA program and had to be at least 15 when they applied, though younger applicants could apply if they were currently in the midst of deportation proceedings. The DACA program also required applicants to be in school, to be a high school graduate or holder of a high school completion certificate or General Education Development (GED), or to be an honorably discharged veteran of the US Armed Forces or Coast Guard. Applicants convicted of a felony, significant misdemeanor, or 3 or more misdemeanors were ineligible for the program. The DACA program recipients have been required to reenroll in the program every 2 years. Enrollment in the DACA program permits the opportunity to receive employment authorization. Deferred action did not grant permanent resident status to approved applicants, nor did it provide a path to citizenship. It also did not convey lawful status to an individual. As of January 2018, most of the individuals

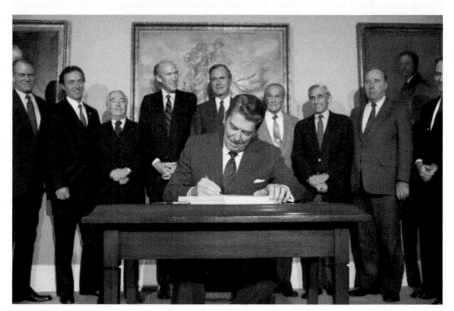

Fig. 6. President Reagan signs into law the Immigration Reform and Control Act of 1986. (*From* Ronald Reagan Presidential Library. Available at: https://www.reaganlibrary.gov/photo-galleries/signing-ceremonies.)

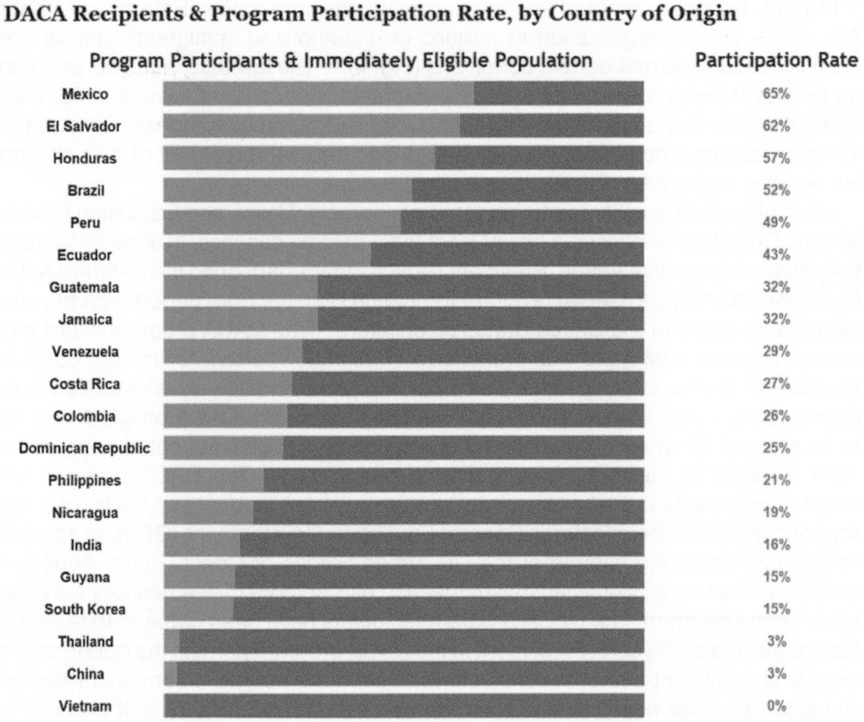

DACA Recipients & Program Participation Rate, by Country of Origin

Program Participants & Immediately Eligible Population	Participation Rate
Mexico	65%
El Salvador	62%
Honduras	57%
Brazil	52%
Peru	49%
Ecuador	43%
Guatemala	32%
Jamaica	32%
Venezuela	29%
Costa Rica	27%
Colombia	26%
Dominican Republic	25%
Philippines	21%
Nicaragua	19%
India	16%
Guyana	15%
South Korea	15%
Thailand	3%
China	3%
Vietnam	0%

Fig. 7. The Migration Policy Institute analysis of the approximate percentage of active recipients of the DACA program as of January 31, 2018. (*Data from* US Citizenship and Immigration Services. Available at: www.uscis.gov/sites/default/files/USCIS/Resources/Reports%20and%20Studies/Immigration%20Forms%20Data/All%20Form%20Types/DACA/DACA_Population_Data_Jan_31_2018.pdf.)

enrolled in the DACA program were those born in Mexico (544,000 of 640,000 eligible Mexican born individuals). All told, by that time, the DACA program had protected more than 800,000 young adults from deportation. The Migration Policy Institute provides estimates of the numbers of enrollees in the DACA program (**Fig. 7**). In September 2017, The US Attorney General announced that the DACA program would come to an end unless Congress passed legislation enacting it. This announcement stopped the program from accepting new applications and would not have allowed anyone whose permit expired after March 6, 2018, to reenroll. In early 2018, a federal judge ruled that the DACA program must remain in place as the legality of the Executive Action in establishing the DACA program is winding its way through the appeals courts. The US Supreme Court has declined to take up a key case dealing with the DACA program, indicating that the lower courts should hear the case first.

SUMMARY

The landscape of US immigration law and policy is ever changing. Until Congress enacts a comprehensive immigration reform bill, it is likely that the patchwork of executive actions and temporary immigration policies will continue. For example, as the legality of the executive order establishing the DACA program was being reviewed in the courts, President Trump signed an executive order that immediately barred entry into the United States for the citizens of Iran, Iraq, Libya, Somalia, Sudan, Syria, and Yemen. The order, dubbed Protection of the Nation from Foreign Terrorist Entry into the United States, also halted the US refugee program for 120 days; however, it indefinitely barred all Syrian refugees from entering the country.[17] In response to legal challenges, the ban was revised twice and, in the end, the Supreme Court upheld the ban.

Since enactment of the INA of 1965, which opened the doors of the country to the diverse populations that now make the United States their home, the needs of minors have for too long been caught up in the overall complexity of immigration policy. Recognition of the unique needs of minors and those of the so-called DACA Dreamers should be addressed as part of comprehensive immigration reform and, if this is not possible, in a more targeted set of legislative proposals. James A. Stockman III's article, "International Migration and Immigration Issues Related to the United States: Defining the Size and Scope of the Problem," which follows discusses the challenges that accompanied and unaccompanied minors face when attempting to enter the country.

REFERENCES

1. Clark U, Dyke P, Shakun A, et al. The last glacial maximum. Science 2009;325: 710–4.
2. Goebel T, Waters MR, O'Rourke DH. The late Pleistocene dispersal of modern humans in the Americas. Science 2008;319:1497–502.
3. History Staff. Puritan history. Available at: History.com http://www.history.com/topics/puritanism. Accessed August 22, 2018.
4. Editor. African American History Timeline: 1701-1800. Available at: http://www.blackpast.org/timelines/african-american-history-timeline-1700-1800. Accessed August 22, 2018.
5. Editor. National Geographic. Meet the 19th century political party founded on ethnic hate. Available at: https://www.nationalgeographic.com/archaeology-and-history/magazine/2017/07-08/know-nothings-and-nativism/. Accessed August 22, 2018.
6. Luo L. The History of Chinese Immigration to the U.S. KCC Alterna-TV News. Available at: http://www2.hawaii.edu/~sford/alternatv/s05/articles/leo_history.html. Accessed August 22,2018.
7. Kanazawa M. Immigration, exclusion, and taxation: anti-Chinese legislation in gold rush California. J Econ Hist 2005;65:779–805.
8. Glass A. Politico. Congress approves first U.S. immigration law, March 26, 1790. Available at: https://www.politico.com/story/2017/03/congress-approves-first-us-immigration-law-march-26-1790-236359. Accessed August 27, 2018.
9. Orth P. The alien contract labor. Polit Sci Quart 1907;22:49–60. Available at: https://www.jstor.org/stable/2140911.
10. Editor. Immigration Act of 1882. Immigration to the United States. Available at: http://immigrationtounitedstates.org/584-immigration-act-of-1882.html. Accessed August 22, 2018.
11. Weisberger M. LiveScience. 'Immigration Act of 1917' Turns 100: America's Long History of Immigration Prejudice. Available at: https://www.livescience.com/57756-1917-immigration-act-100th-anniversary.html. Accessed August 27, 2018.
12. Editor. Office of the Historian, US Government. The Immigration Act of 1924 (The Johnson-Reed Act). Available at: https://history.state.gov/milestones/1921-1936/immigration-act. Accessed August 18, 2018.

13. Editor. The Immigration and Nationality Act of 1952 (The McCarran-Walter Act). Office of the Historian, US Government. Available at: https://history.state.gov/milestones/1945-1952/immigration-act. Accessed August 30, 2018.

14. History Staff. History. U.S. Immigration Since 1965. Available at: https://www.history.com/topics/us-immigration-since-1965. Accessed August 27, 2018.

15. U.S. Citizenship and Immigration Services Staff. USCIS. Immigration Reform and Control Act of 1986 (IRCA). Available at: https://www.uscis.gov/tools/glossary/immigration-reform-and-control-act-1986-irca. Accessed August 27, 2018.

16. USCIS Staff. USCIS. Consideration of Deferred Action for Childhood Arrivals (DACA). Available at: https://www.uscis.gov/archive/consideration-deferred-action-childhood-arrivals-daca. Accessed August 27,2018.

17. Barnes R, Marimow AE. Washington Post. Supreme Court Upholds Trump Travel Ban. Available at: https://www.washingtonpost.com/politics/courts_law/supreme-court-upholds-trump-travel-ban/2018/06/26/b79cb09a-7943-11e8-80be-6d32e182a3bc_story.html?utm_term=.5550105c3762. Accessed August 29, 2018.

International Migration and Immigration Issues Related to the United States
Defining the Size and Scope of the Problem

James A. Stockman III, MD

KEYWORDS

- International migration • Refugees • Asylum
- US Citizenship and Immigration Services (USCIS)
- The Immigration and Customs Enforcement (ICE) • Customs and Border Patrol (CBP)

KEY POINTS

- The provision of immigration services has been less than adequate.
- The numbers of refugees worldwide are approximately twice that seen 10 years ago. According to United Nations High Commissioner for Refugees, if measured against the world's population of 7.4 billion people, 1 in every 122 people globally is now either an asylum seeker, internally displaced, or a refugee.
- Oversight and implementation of immigration policy in the United States is ever changing but currently is carried out principally by 3 federal agencies that were formed after 9/11. The 3 agencies are the US Citizenship and Immigration Services, the Immigration and Customs Enforcement, and Customs and Border Patrol.
- Due to their vulnerability, migrant children, particularly those who are unaccompanied, are entitled to receive certain additional protections under US law.

INTRODUCTION

The past several years has seen more displaced families and individuals than in the past half century. This in part is the result of ongoing conflicts occurring in Syria, Afghanistan, Somalia, and to a lesser extent in Central America, in particular, Honduras, Guatemala, and El Salvador. The impact on the immigration, health, and social services of the countries receiving displaced persons has been enormous. In many instances, the provision of immigration services has been less than adequate.

This article briefly examines the scope of international migration–related issues. Also covered are issues related to the migration of individuals and families across

Disclosure Statement: Author has nothing to disclose.
American Board of Pediatrics, 111 Silver Cedar Court, Chapel Hill, NC 27514, USA
E-mail address: jstockman@abpeds.org

Pediatr Clin N Am 66 (2019) 537–547
https://doi.org/10.1016/j.pcl.2019.02.003
0031-3955/19/© 2019 Elsevier Inc. All rights reserved.

pediatric.theclinics.com

the southern border of this country. For the purposes of definition, *migrant* is defined as an adult, child, or family unit that moves within or beyond national borders, usually with sociocultural, educational, or economic motives, rather than being forcibly uprooted. *Refugees* are persons that are outside their home country because of a well-founded fear of being persecuted or in flight from the threat of armed conflict. An *asylum seeker* (an "asylee") is a person who has arrived in another country and has sought protection.

INTERNATIONAL MIGRATION: THE OVERALL PICTURE

The Office of the United Nations High Commissioner for Refugees (UNHCR), launched in 1950 and known as the "UN Refugee Agency," is a United Nations program mandated to protect and support refugees.[1] Current information provided by UNHCR indicates that there are 68.5 million forcibly displaced people worldwide, including 40 million that are displaced internally within their own country.[2] Of these, 25 million are considered refugees by the UNHCR. More than half of these refugees are younger than 18 years. In addition, 3.1 million are asylum seekers. There are also an estimated 10 million stateless people who have been denied a nationality and access to basic rights such as education, health care, employment, and freedom of movement.

The numbers of refugees worldwide are approximately twice that seen 10 years ago. According to UNHCR, if measured against the world's population of 7.4 billion people, 1 in every 122 people globally is now an asylum seeker, internally displaced, or a refugee. This is a number greater than the population of some developed nations.

Of refugees worldwide, 57% come from just 3 countries: South Sudan (2.4 million), Afghanistan (2.6 million), and Syria (6.3 million). Of all displaced people, 85% are being housed in developing countries throughout the Middle East and, to a lesser extent, Europe and elsewhere (including the United States). **Fig. 1** illustrates the 5 major countries that have accepted displaced individuals and families over the past several years.

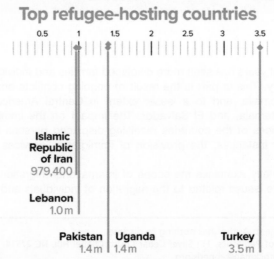

Fig. 1. Placement of displaced individuals and families. United Nations Human Rights Council June 19, 2018. (*From* the United Nations High Commissioner for Refugees. Figures at a Glance; with permission. Available at: http://www.unhcr.org/en-us/figures-at-a-glance. html. Accessed March 20, 2019.)

IMMIGRATION ISSUES RELATED TO THE UNITED STATES

Several immigration issues are common to most countries. One is how to design oversight policies that are consistent with international treaties yet are tailored to suit the unique circumstances of recipient countries. The successful integration into the general population of refugees and asylum seekers is another. How to deal with undocumented foreigners who have gained entry across a border is a ubiquitous problem. Most importantly for all countries, ways must be found that allow accompanied and unaccompanied minors to live a full and healthy existence as they wend their way through what is a most difficult time in their lives. These and other challenges to our immigration system must be addressed. What follows are some of these challenges as they relate to the United States.

Oversight and Implementation of United States Immigration Policy

Oversight and implementation of immigration policy in the United States is ever changing but currently is carried out principally by 3 federal agencies that were formed after 9/11. These agencies replaced the Immigration and Naturalization Service in 2002. The 3 agencies are the US Citizenship and Immigration Services (USCIS), the Immigration and Customs Enforcement (ICE), and Customs and Border Patrol (CBP).

Fig. 2, an abbreviated organizational chart, illustrates the 3 Federal Departments that deal with the overall implementation of US immigration policy. They are the Department of Homeland Security (DHS), which oversees USCIS, ICE, and CBP; the Department of Health and Human Services (HHS), which oversees the Office of Refugee Resettlement (ORR); and the Justice Department, which oversees immigration courts.

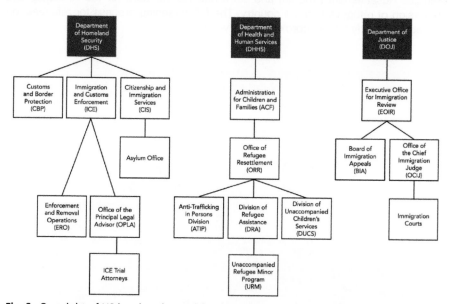

Fig. 2. Oversight of US immigration activity. (*From* Byrne O, Miller E. The flow of unaccompanied children through the immigration system. New York: Vera Institute of Justice. Available at: http://immigrantchildren.org/PDF/03-01-12%20the-flow-of-unaccompanied-children-through-the-immigration-system%20copy.pdf. Accessed March 20, 2019; with permission.)

The regulatory oversight of this country's immigration policy goes back many years. The Immigration Act of 1891 established an Office of the Superintendent of Immigration within the Treasury Department. With this Act, the federal government assumed the ultimate direct control of inspecting, admitting, rejecting, and processing all immigrants seeking admission to the United States. Previously, many states had set their own policies for foreigners. A year later, the Immigration Service opened Ellis Island in New York Harbor (**Fig. 3**). Ellis Island was the gateway for more than 12 million immigrants to the United States. From 1892 to 1954 when it was closed, Ellis Island was the country's busiest immigrant inspection station. The enormous facility housed inspection operations, hearing and detention rooms, hospitals, cafeterias, administrative offices, railroad ticket offices, and the representatives of many immigrant aid societies. Ellis Island station employed 119 of the Immigration Service's entire staff of 180 in 1893. The Service built additional immigrant stations at other principal ports of entry through the early twentieth century. USCIS now oversees lawful immigration to the United States and naturalization of new American citizens. On the heels of the Reed-Johnson Act of 1924, and in response to rising numbers of illegal entries and alien smuggling, especially along land borders, Congress created the CBP. The current CBP is charged with preventing drugs, weapons, terrorists, and other inadmissible persons from entering the country. The role of ICE is to enforce criminal and civil laws governing border control, customs, trade, and immigration.

Refugees

Of those foreign-born individuals who have entered the country legally, approximately 3 million that had been identified as refugees have been resettled in the United States since Congress passed the Refugee Act of 1980.[3] This Act created the Federal Refugee Resettlement Program and set a national standard for the screening and admission of refugees into the country. The full screening process for refugees, on average, currently takes approximately 2 years.

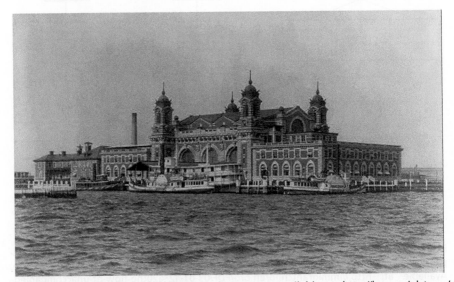

Fig. 3. Ellis Island (1905). (*From* Library of Congress. Available at: http://loc.gov/pictures/resource/cph.3a38144/. Accessed March 20, 2019.)

The total number of refugees presenting to the United States has fluctuated along with global events and US priorities. In the early 1990s, an average of approximately 112,000 refugees arrived in the United States each year, with many coming from countries of the former Soviet Union. By 2002, refugee admissions dropped to fewer than 27,000. This was following the terrorist attacks in Washington, DC, and New York City on September 11, 2001. The refugee number has since trended upward again. In 2016, the highest number of refugees entering the United States came from the Democratic Republic of Congo (16,370) followed by Syria (12,587), Burma, aka Myanmar (12,347), Iraq (9880), and Somalia (9020). Muslims made up nearly half (46%) of all refugee admissions, a higher share than for Christians (44%).[4] Overall, nearly 39,000 Muslim refugees entered the United States in 2016, the highest number on record.

Although the United States did meet its goal of accepting 10,000 Syrian refugees in 2016, by comparison, in the same year, Canada had resettled 25,000 Syrian refugees. Since 2011, Germany has received more than 300,000 asylum petitions. Sweden has taken in more than 100,000 refugees in the past 5 years. As noted previously, the greatest burden has been carried by Turkey, Lebanon, and Jordan. Turkey has hosted more than 2.7 million Syrian refugees, more than any other country. Lebanon has absorbed more than 1 million, whereas Jordan has taken in more than 650,000 refugees. With the US administration's 2017 ban on accepting refugees from several Muslim countries, it was anticipated that the overall numbers of refugees entering the United States was expected to fall dramatically in 2018.

Undocumented Foreigners in the United States

Of the foreign-born residing legally in this country, 19 million are naturalized US citizens. Another 12 million are lawful immigrants, and roughly 2 million are lawful temporary visitors, including students and guest workers.[5] Undocumented foreigners account for a quarter of the 44 million foreign-born residing in the United States. The number of undocumented foreigners rose rapidly from the 1990s through the mid-2000s, peaking at 12 million in 2007 before declining during and after the 2008 to 2009 recession.

Although there are an estimated 20 million lawful foreign-born workers in this country, some 8 million undocumented foreigners are in the US labor force. They comprise approximately 5% of the workforce. Undocumented workers account for a significant component of the workforce in many parts of the country. For example, more than 50% of fruit pickers in California are undocumented foreigners.

Movement of Minors Across the United States Southern Border

Children who enter the country are broadly classified as being "accompanied" or "unaccompanied." Accompanied children are those who on presentation are with a family member, a responsible adult, or a guardian. Accompanied children are, in general, covered under the standard immigration policies dealing with entry of families. An "unaccompanied alien child" is a technical term defined by law as a child who has no lawful immigration status in the United States, has not attained 18 years of age, and who has no parent or legal guardian in this country to provide care and physical custody. Most unaccompanied minors are teenage boys ages 14 to 17.[6]

Over the past several years, increasing numbers of children and their families have been fleeing violence in Guatemala, Honduras, and El Salvador, a region of Central America known as the "Northern Triangle." Researchers consistently cite increased violence in the Northern Triangle as the primary motivation for this migration. Poverty and a desire for family reunification are among the other causes. In 2016, the migration of unaccompanied minors to the US southern borders mostly consisted of children from El Salvador (17,512) Guatemala (18,913), and Honduras (10,468). Some also come from Mexico. By 2017, the overall number of unaccompanied children presenting to our southern boarders was 41,435.[7] The CBP reported that in the first half of 2018, 37,450 apprehensions of unaccompanied children had taken place.[8] Almost all are turning themselves over to Border Patrol agents and are not seeking to evade apprehension[9]

United States Immigration Protections for Minors

The United States has entered treaties with other countries to ensure the protection and safe passage of refugees. Among the most important are the 1951 United Nations Convention Relating to the Status of Refugees. The Convention has been signed by 145 states. The UNHCR serves as the "guardian" of the 1951 Convention and its 1967 Protocol.[10] Under these United Nations treaties, the United States may not return an individual to a country where he or she faces persecution from a government or a group the government is unable or unwilling to control based on race, religion, nationality, political opinion, or membership in a social group. A separate treaty, known as the Convention Against Torture, prohibits the return of people to a country where there are substantial grounds to believe they may be tortured.[11] More than 50% of the children who the UNHCR has surveyed from Honduras, El Salvador, and Guatemala appear to qualify as international refugees. Moreover, children may qualify for humanitarian relief as victims of trafficking and crime, or as children who have been abused or abandoned by their parents.

Because of their vulnerability, migrant children, particularly those who are unaccompanied, receive certain additional protections under US law. A 2-decade-old court case, the *Flores* settlement[12] and a law called the Trafficking Victims Protection Reauthorization Act (TVPRA) both specify how the government must treat migrant children.[13] They require that migrant children be placed in "the least restrictive environment" or sent to live with family members. They also limit how long families with children can be detained; courts have interpreted that limit as 20 days.

Most unaccompanied children encountered at the border are apprehended, processed, and initially detained by CBP. Unlike adults or children in families, unaccompanied children cannot be placed into expedited removal proceedings. Children from noncontiguous countries, such as El Salvador, Guatemala, and Honduras, are placed into standard removal proceedings in immigration court. CBP must transfer custody of these children to HHS and its ORR within 72 hours. Accompanied children and adults from a contiguous country (Mexico or Canada) may be returned promptly to their home countries. Unaccompanied children from Mexico or Canada, however, must be screened by a CBP officer to determine if he or she is unable to make independent decisions, is a victim of trafficking, or fears persecution in his home country. If none of these conditions apply, CBP may send the child back to Mexico or Canada through a process called "voluntary return." Return occurs pursuant to agreements with Mexico and Canada to manage the repatriation process. Nongovernmental organizations have expressed concern in the strongest of terms that CBP is the "wrong agency" to screen children for signs of trauma, abuse, or persecution.

It should be noted that many minors never make it to the southern border of the United States. If identified by Mexican authorities, Mexican border officials may directly return minors to their home countries in Central America. Deportations from Mexico to the Northern Triangle countries have increased significantly over the past decade. According to a Pew Research Center analysis of data from the Mexican government, Mexico deported 3819 unaccompanied minors from Central America during the first 5 months of 2015, a 56% increase over the same period from 2014. Unfortunately, children who are deported in such a manner may not always undergo thorough screening, including for trafficking, as required by international law.[14]

As noted, unaccompanied children must be transferred from the DHS to the custody of HHS within 72 hours of apprehension. ORR then manages the custody and care of the children until they can be released to family members or other individuals or organizations while their court proceedings go forward. Under the TVPRA, HHS is required to "promptly place" each child in its custody "in the least restrictive setting that is in the best interests of the child." As such, children in ORR care are generally housed through a network of state-licensed, ORR-funded care providers, who are tasked with providing educational, health, and case management services to children. Placement may include a parent, a legal guardian, an adult relative, an adult individual or entity designated by the child's parent or legal guardian, a licensed program willing to accept legal custody, or an adult or entity approved by ORR. The sponsor must agree to ensure that the child attends immigration court.

Over the first 9 years of ORR's operation, fewer than 8000 children were served annually in this program. In 2016, the program received 59,170 unaccompanied minor referrals. Approximately half of all unaccompanied children who were referred to ORR were 14 years or older and two-thirds were boys. In 2017, the countries of origin for these youth were Guatemala (45%), El Salvador (27%), Honduras (23%), and other (3%). Currently, the average length of stay for unaccompanied minors in the ORR program is approximately 57 days.[15] Under international law, children should in principle not be detained at all according to UNHCR Resolution 57.[16] UNHCR Resolution 57 recognizes that detention has well-documented negative effects on children's mental and physical development, especially when it is indefinite in nature.

Access to Counsel by Unaccompanied Minors

Among the most common types of US immigration relief that children might potentially have available to them are the following, all of which require the advice of counsel given the complexity of the various laws and regulations associated with them:

- Asylum: Asylum is a form of international protection granted to refugees who are present in the United States. To qualify for asylum, a child or adult must demonstrate a well-founded fear of persecution based on 1 of 5 grounds: race, religion, nationality, political opinion, or membership in a social group.
- Special Immigrant Juvenile Status (SIJS): SIJS is a humanitarian form of relief available to noncitizen minors who were abused, neglected, or abandoned by 1 or both parents. To be eligible for SIJS, a child must be younger than 21, unmarried, and the subject of certain dependency orders issued by a juvenile court.
- U visas: A U visa is available to victims of certain crimes. To be eligible, the person must have suffered substantial physical or mental abuse and have cooperated with law enforcement in the investigation or prosecution of the crime.
- T visas: A T visa is available to individuals who have been victims of a severe form of trafficking. To be eligible, the person must demonstrate that he or she would suffer extreme hardship involving unusual or severe harm if removed from the United States.

Unfortunately, minors may not always be aware of the protections available to them including options regarding appeals to deportation. Children facing deportation, just like adults facing deportation, are not provided government-appointed counsel to represent them in immigration court. Under current immigration law, all persons have the *"privilege"* of being represented *"at no expense to the government."*[17] This means that only those individuals who can afford a private lawyer or those who are able to find pro bono counsel to represent them free of charge are represented in immigration court.

Pro bono legal service providers are unable to meet the need of all immigrant children. Many are left without counsel to effectively mount a defense against a government attorney arguing for deportation. Government data indicate that, of all cases from 2005 through May 2018, half of juveniles in deportation proceedings were not represented by an attorney.[18] These include more than 38,000 cases of minors. In such instances, children are forced to appear before an immigration judge and must navigate the immigration court process, including putting on a legal defense, without any legal representation. In contrast, DHS, which acts as the prosecutor in immigration court and argues for the child's deportation, is represented in every case by a lawyer trained in immigration law. Some of the children undergoing deportation review who have been without counsel in recent times were just a few years of age.

The American Immigration Council filed a nationwide class-action lawsuit challenging the federal government's failure to provide children with legal representation in immigration court. The case, *JEFM v. Holder*, entered the judicial system in 2014.[19] The complaint charges the US Department of Justice, DHS, HHS, Department of Health and Executive Office for Immigration Review, and ORR with violating the US Constitution's Fifth Amendment Due Process Clause and the Immigration and Nationality Act's provisions requiring a "full and fair hearing" before an immigration judge. The suit seeks to require the government to provide children with legal representation in their deportation hearings.

As of the summer of 2018, immigrant children subject to deportation or asylum hearings are still not entitled to court-appointed lawyers. Currently, no defendant of any age is provided with court-appointed attorneys in immigration court because they are not technically accused of crimes. Civil offenses are not covered under the US Constitution. The Vera Institute of Justice estimates that 40% of immigrant children unaccompanied by a parent or guardian are eligible for some form of relief from deportation.[20] Without question, representation by legal counsel is of advantage to children facing deportation. In all deportation hearings over the past 5 years, children with attorneys won 85% of the time.[21] Those without legal counsel lost 87% of the time.

The Problem of Separation of Children from Families

Before 2006, ICE commonly detained parents and children separately. In 2006, however, Congress directed ICE to either "release families," use "alternatives to detention such as the Intensive Supervised Appearance Program," or, if necessary, use "appropriate" detention space to house families together.[22] Despite this, on May 8, 2018, Attorney General Jeff Sessions announced that for immigrants illegally crossing borders, officials would enforce a "zero-tolerance policy" explicitly stating that one effect of the policy would be the enforced separation of children from their parents. Multiple administration officials justified such a move on the grounds that this forced separation could serve as a deterrent to future illegal immigration. Before this zero-tolerance policy was in widespread use, CBP had significantly more leeway in deciding which cases they referred for prosecution, thus limiting the number of family units that would have been separated before referring them to ORR. Between May 5, 2018, and June 9, 2018, 2342 children were separated from 2206 parents at the US-Mexico border, and with no apparent plan for reuniting them with their families. On June 18, 2018, following widespread bipartisan and international condemnation of the "zero-tolerance policy," the administration reversed course, attempting to fix the separation issue with a vague (and somewhat ineffective) Executive Order.

PHYSICAL AND EMOTIONAL CONSEQUENCES OF DISPLACEMENT

Studies, mostly from abroad, of detained immigrants have found numerous negative physical and emotional symptoms among detained children, including posttraumatic symptoms that do not always disappear at the time of release.[23] Young detainees may experience developmental delay and poor psychological adjustment, potentially affecting functioning in school. Qualitative reports about detained unaccompanied immigrant children in the United States have found high rates of posttraumatic stress disorder, anxiety, depression, suicidal ideation, and other behavioral problems.[24]

The conditions (eg, famine, poverty, war) that migrants face before the start of their journey from their homeland may also have long lasting effects. The journeys are hardly risk free. For example, children from Central America arriving unaccompanied to the United States must travel by land through Mexico, a notoriously dangerous undertaking. Middle Eastern and African minors arriving in the European Union sometimes have traveled by land, but more often make perilous journeys in rickety boats crossing the Mediterranean Sea. Thousands never make it to their destination. During these journeys, girl migrants have a higher likelihood of exposure to rapes and sexual violence, by smugglers, authorities, and criminals alike.[25] Migrants are commonly exposed to assaults, robberies, torture, inhumane treatment, sexual violence, and even death. According to Amnesty International, 6 of 10 Central American women and girls are victims of sexual violence during their journey through Mexico.[26]

With respect to detention, there is no evidence indicating that any time in detention is safe for children. Two years before the "zero-tolerance" policy was announced in the Spring of 2018, the DHS Advisory Committee on Family Residential Centers had issued a report on the detention of immigrants.[27] The Report made very specific recommendations that included the statement that detention or the separation of families for purposes of immigration enforcement or management is *never* in the best interest of children. The report additionally recommended that the DHS should discontinue the general use of family detention, reserving it for rare cases when necessary following an individualized assessment of the need to detain because of danger or flight risk that cannot be mitigated by conditions of release and that if such an assessment determines that continued custody is absolutely necessary, families should be detained for the shortest amount of time and in the least restrictive setting possible.

SUMMARY

The UNHCR will continue to hold countries that have signed onto international agreements on refugees to the commitments they have made to deal with current and future immigration crises. Here in the United States, until there is comprehensive immigration reform that acknowledges the unique issues of displaced children, we are likely to continue to see the emotional and physical consequences of our poorly designed immigration policies.

Linton and colleagues[28] have summarized many aspects of the current US immigration processes that affect children attempting to enter the country, either as unaccompanied minors or as part of a family unit. The summary of Linton and colleagues[28] also provides guidelines for the care of immigrant children, particularly those who may be exhibiting the adverse medical and psychological consequences of displacements and possible detention. Both the American Academy of Pediatrics and the Centers for Disease Control and Prevention have also provided excellent resources for primary care providers to use when caring for immigrant children.[29,30] Every pediatric care provider should become familiar with these resources.

REFERENCES

1. UNHRC. UNHRC USA. Home page. Available at: http://www.unhcr.org/en-us/. Accessed August 25, 2018.
2. UNHR Staff. UNHR. Figures at a glance. Available at: http://www.unhcr.org/en-us/figures-at-a-glance.html. Accessed August 23, 2018.
3. National Archives Foundation. The National Archives. The Refugee Act of 1980. Available at: https://www.archivesfoundation.org/documents/refugee-act-1980/. Accessed August 25, 2018.
4. Capps R, Fix M. Ten facts about U.S. Refugee Resettlement. Migration Policy Institute. Available at: https://www.migrationpolicy.org/. Accessed August 25, 2018.
5. Brown A, Stepler R. Pew Research Center. How many undocumented?. Available at: http://www.pewhispanic.org/2002/03/21/how-many-undocumented/. Accessed August 27, 2018.
6. Hunter A, Shklyan K. Pew Charitable Trust. Unaccompanied minors—the state and local story. Washington, DC. Available at: http://www.pewtrusts.org/en/research-and-analysis/blogs/stateline/2016/04/14/unaccompanied-minors-the-stateand-local-story. Accessed August 23, 2018.
7. U.S. Customs and Immigration. Statistics. U.S. Border Patrol Southwest Border Apprehensions by Sector. FY2017 Southwest Border Unaccompanied Alien Children (0-17 yr. old) Apprehensions. Available at: https://www.cbp.gov/newsroom/stats/sw-border-migration-fy2017. Accessed August 26, 2018.
8. U.S. Customs and Immigration. Statistics. Southwest Border Migration FY2018. Available at: https://www.cbp.gov/newsroom/stats/sw-border-migration. Accessed August 26, 2018.
9. Beltrán A. WOLA. Statement before Congressional progressive caucus on protecting children fleeing violence: examining the southern border humanitarian crisis 2014. Available at: https://www.wola.org/analysis/wolas-adriana-beltrans-testimony-before-the-congressionalprogressive- caucus/. Accessed August 27, 2018.
10. UNHRC Staff. UNHRC. United Nations convention relating to the status of refugees and related protocol. Available at: http://www.unhcr.org/en-us/3b66c2aa10. Accessed August 26, 2018.
11. Committee on Human Rights, United Nations. Convention against torture and other cruel, inhuman or degrading treatment or punishment. Available at: https://www.ohchr.org/en/professionalinterest/pages/CAT.aspx. Accessed August 26, 2018.
12. ACLU Staff. ACLU. Flores v. Meese - stipulated settlement agreement plus extension of settlement. Available at: https://www.aclu.org/legal-document/flores-v-meese-stipulated-settlement-agreement-plus-extension-settlement. Accessed August 26, 2018.
13. US State Department Staff. United States Department of State. U.S. laws on trafficking in persons. Available at: https://www.state.gov/j/tip/laws/. Accessed August 26, 2018.
14. Pew Foundation Staff. Pew Research Foundation. Q&A: unaccompanied children from Central America, one year later. Available at: http://www.pewtrusts.org/en/research-and-analysis/blogs/stateline/2015/08/24/unaccompanied-children-from-central-america-one-year-later. Accessed August 26, 2018.

15. ORR Staff. HHS. Fact sheet, unaccompanied children. Available at: https://www. acf.hhs.gov/sites/default/files/orr/orr_fact_sheet_on_unaccompanied_alien_ childrens_services_0.pdf. Accessed August 26. 2018.
16. UN Staff. UNHRC. Immigration Bill 2015-16/Briefing on Amendments 57; 84 and 116A. Available at: http://www.unhcr.org/en-us/protection/basic/57515d9c4/ immigration-bill-amendments-57-84-and-116a-unhcr-parliamentary-briefing.html. Accessed August 26, 2018.
17. Eagly I, Shafer S. American Immigration Counsel. Special Report. Access to counsel in immigration court. Available at: https://www.americanimmigrationcouncil.org/ research/access-counsel-immigration-court. Accessed August 27, 2018.
18. TRAC Immigration. Juvenile Court Cases. Juveniles — immigration court deportation proceedings. Available at: http://trac.syr.edu/phptools/immigration/ juvenile/. Accessed August 27, 2018.
19. ACLU Staff. ACLU. J.E.F.M. v. Holder – complaint. Available at: https://www.aclu. org/legal-document/jefm-v-holder-complaint. Accessed August 27, 2018.
20. Mulcahy AM. Vera Institute. Legal services for unaccompanied children. Available at: https://www.vera.org/projects/legal-services-for-unaccompanied-children. Accessed August 27, 2018.
21. Zoukis C. Prison Legal News. Federal judge claims three-year-olds can understand immigration law. Available at: https://www.prisonlegalnews.org/news/ 2017/aug/29/federal-judge-claims-three-year-olds-can-understand-immigration-law/. Accessed August 27, 2018.
22. Staff Report. American Immigration Council. A guide to children arriving at the border: laws, policies and responses. Available at: https://www. americanimmigrationcouncil.org/research/guide-children-arriving-border-laws-policies-and-responses. Accessed August 27, 2018.
23. Robjant K, Hassan R, Katona C. Mental health implications of detaining asylum seekers: systematic review. Br J Psychiatry 2009;194(4):306–12.
24. Bailey C, Henderson SW, Taub AR, et al. The mental health needs of unaccompanied immigrant children: lawyers' role as a conduit to services. Graduate Student Journal of Psychology 2014;15:3–17. Available at: https://www.tc.columbia.edu/ publications/gsjp/gsjp-volumes-archive/36302_1baileyetal.pdf.
25. Parish A. Migration Policy Institute. Gender-based violence against women: both cause for migration and risk along the journey. Available at: https://www. migrationpolicy.org/article/gender-based-violence-against-women-both-cause-migration-and-risk-along-journey. Accessed August 27, 2018.
26. Pereira F. El Mundo. Cruzar México, un infierno para los centroamericanos." La Nación. Available at: http://www.lanacion.com.ar/1280709-cruzar-mexico-un-infiernopara- los-centroamericanos. Accessed August 27, 2018.
27. DHS Staff. DHS. Report of the DHS Advisory Committee on Family Residential Centers. 2016. Available at: https://www.ice.gov/sites/default/files/documents/ Report/2016/ACFRC-sc-16093.pdf. Accessed August 27, 2018.
28. Linton JM, Griffin M, Shapiro AJ, et al. Detention of immigrant children. Pediatrics 2017;139(5) [pii:e20170483].
29. American Academy of Pediatrics. Trauma toolbox for primary care. Elk Grove Village (IL): American Academy of Pediatrics; 2014. Available at: https://www. aap.org/en-us/advocacy-and-policy/aap-health-initiatives/Immigrant-Child-Health-Toolkit/Pages/Immigrant-Child-Health-Toolkit.aspx. Accessed August 27, 2018.
30. CDC Staff. CDC. Guidelines for the U.S. domestic medical examination for newly arriving refugees. Available at: https://www.cdc.gov/immigrantrefugeehealth/ guidelines/domestic/domestic-guidelines.html. Accessed August 24, 2018.

Immigrant and Refugee Health

A Centers for Disease Control and Prevention Perspective on Protecting the Health and Health Security of Individuals and Communities During Planned Migrations

Tarissa Mitchell, MD*, Michelle Weinberg, MD, MPH, Drew L. Posey, MD, MPH, Martin Cetron, MD

KEYWORDS

- Migration • Emigrants and immigrants • Refugees • Vaccination • Tuberculosis
- Parasitic diseases • Health care costs • Centers for Disease Control and Prevention

KEY POINTS

- With global forced displacement and migration at record levels, it is critical to ensure both the health of migrating populations and the health security of receiving countries.
- Based on 22 years of experience in development and monitoring of a health assessment framework for US-bound immigrants and refugees, the Centers for Disease Control and Prevention's Division of Global Migration and Quarantine has identified successful strategies to improve health during planned migrations, including overseas screening, treatment, and vaccination programs.
- These strategies have reduced US tuberculosis rates; decreased transmission and importation of vaccine-preventable diseases; prevented morbidity from parasitic diseases; and saved domestic health costs.
- This approach to screening, treatment, and prevention represents one important health model in the planned migration setting.

Disclosure Statement: Drs T. Mitchell, M. Weinberg, D.L. Posey, and M. Cetron have no financial relationships to disclose.
Disclaimer: The findings and conclusions in this report are those of the authors and do not necessarily represent the official position of CDC.
Centers for Disease Control and Prevention, 1600 Clifton Road NE, MS E-03, Atlanta, GA 30333, USA
* Corresponding author.
E-mail address: TMitchell1@cdc.gov

Pediatr Clin N Am 66 (2019) 549–560
https://doi.org/10.1016/j.pcl.2019.02.004
0031-3955/19/Published by Elsevier Inc. This is an open access article under the CC BY-NC-ND license (http://creativecommons.org/licenses/by-nc-nd/4.0/).

pediatric.theclinics.com

With more than 1 billion people crossing international borders each year and dramatic increases in the speed of global travel,[1] there is nowhere remote in the world, and no one from whom we are disconnected. Current trends in human migration illustrate this reality. Defined as persons changing their country of usual residence,[2] most migrants make a choice to move, although for many, poverty and necessity are the major reasons behind that choice. However, the world is also seeing record levels of forced migration and displacement resulting from an unparalleled number of simultaneous, complex, and protracted crises involving armed conflicts, political upheavals, natural disasters, climate change, and human rights deprivation.

Indeed, by United Nations High Commissioner for Refugees (UNHCR) estimates, there were 68.5 million forcibly displaced people worldwide by the end of 2017. Of these, 25.4 million were refugees, the highest number ever. More than half were children younger than 18 years old.[3] Refugees, as defined in the 1951 Geneva Convention, are persons outside their country of nationality who are unable or unwilling to return because of a well-founded fear of persecution based on race, religion, nationality, membership in a social group, or political opinion.[4] Numbers are swelling in the context of wars and political unrest in countries such as Syria, Iraq, Afghanistan, the Democratic Republic of the Congo, and Somalia; and of the persecution facing ethnic and religious minorities in Burma and other countries.

Many refugees seek asylum in nearby countries. For example, in 2016, asylum countries with the highest number of refugees included Turkey, Jordan, the Palestinian Territories, Lebanon, and Pakistan.[5] Fewer than 1% of all refugees become eligible for resettlement to a third country, when limited prospects exist for either returning home or remaining permanently in the country of asylum.[6] These refugees are identified by UNHCR and referred as applicants to countries participating in UNHCR's resettlement program, including the United States, which has hosted a Refugee Admissions Program (USRAP) since 1980.[7]

IMMIGRANTS AND REFUGEES BOUND TO THE UNITED STATES

Historically, the United States has been the world's top resettlement country.[6] The peak year for refugee resettlement to the United States was 1980, when more than 200,000 refugees arrived, mainly from Cambodia and Vietnam. In federal fiscal year (FY) 2018, approximately 20,000 refugees resettled to the United States; **Fig. 1** shows refugees resettled that year by receiving state, with populous states such as California, Texas, and New York among the leading receiving states. The top 5 countries of nationality for US-bound refugees in FY 2018 were the Democratic Republic of the Congo, Burma, Ukraine, Bhutan, and Eritrea,[8] although resettlement numbers and origins may change annually (**Fig. 2**). Still, refugees constitute a tiny proportion of the international travelers arriving on our shores annually. For example, the largest annual number of refugees received in the past 2 decades was approximately 85,000, in FY 2016. This number constituted 0.05% of roughly 180 million US-bound international travelers that same year, including approximately 1 million immigrants and millions of nonimmigrant admissions, such as tourists, students, and persons on employment visas.[9] The roughly 1.2 million immigrants obtaining lawful permanent residency (LPR) status during that year originated in more than 200 countries and territories; a plurality were born in Asia (approximately 39%) or North America (approximately 36%).[8]

Health assessment represents an important component of the migration process for US-bound immigrants and refugees. These assessments support the health of

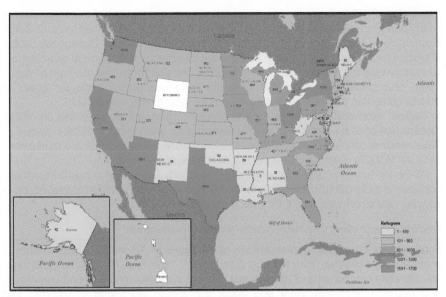

Fig. 1. Refugee arrivals by state, FY 2018. (*Courtesy of* DGMQ/CDC.)

migrating populations as well as US domestic health security, promote collaboration with state and international health partners, and strengthen our understanding of the health profiles of diverse arriving populations. We describe several related programs here.

MEDICAL EXAMINATION OF US-BOUND IMMIGRANTS AND REFUGEES

US-bound immigrants and refugees are required to undergo a medical examination overseas before traveling to the United States. The Centers for Disease Control and

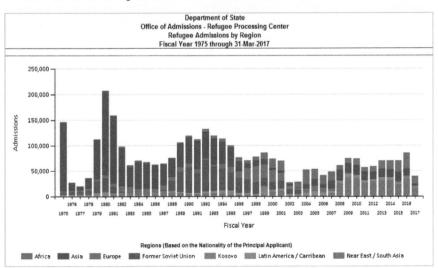

Fig. 2. Origins and numbers of US refugee admissions over time, 1975 to 2017. (*Data from* Refugee Processing Center. Admissions & Arrivals. Available at: http://www.wrapsnet.org/admissions-and-arrivals/. Accessed September 21, 2018.)

Prevention (CDC) is the federal agency with regulatory oversight of this examination, which is performed by panel physicians appointed by the US Department of State. Examinations follow technical instructions provided by CDC's Division of Global Migration and Quarantine (DGMQ) and consist of a history and physical examination; laboratory testing for tuberculosis (TB), syphilis, and gonorrhea; assessment of vaccination status; identification of mental health conditions posing a danger to self or others; screening for substance abuse; and, for immigrants, vaccination.[10]

Medical examination findings and vaccination history are documented on official Department of State forms. For all refugees, and for immigrants with tuberculosis or other medical conditions of public health significance, these records are transmitted to DGMQ/CDC's Electronic Disease Notification system, or EDN.

US-bound immigrants and refugees diagnosed with a condition of public health significance are eligible to come to the United States once the condition is treated, or, in special, rare circumstances, if they have obtained a waiver.

Medical Examination: The Tuberculosis Technical Instructions

Foreign-born TB cases represent 65% of all cases of TB in the United States, a proportion that has risen over the past 2 decades.[11] Therefore, TB detection and treatment are key components of the required medical evaluation of US-bound immigrants and refugees. Between 1999 and 2005, 2.7 million US-bound immigrants and 279,000 US-bound refugees were screened for TB overseas. Previous TB Technical Instructions (TBTI), developed in 1991, required only sputum smears for adult immigrants or refugees with abnormal chest radiographs. However, evidence suggested that sputum cultures could increase diagnostic yield. For example, a study conducted in 1998 to 1999 among US-bound immigrants in Vietnam demonstrated that smear-based screening was only 34% as sensitive as sputum culture, indicating that some active TB cases could be missed using sputum smear alone.[12] Further, a 2009 report indicated that rates of smear-negative, radiograph-positive tuberculosis (eg, chest radiograph suggestive of active TB) were as high as 961 of 100,000.[13] Hence, the TBTI were modified in 2007. Titled "Culture and Directly Observed Therapy TB Technical Instructions," the 2007 instructions call for chest radiographs in all US-bound immigrants and refugees aged ≥15 years along with sputum smear *plus* culture with drug susceptibility testing in those with abnormal radiograph findings, and for anyone with human immunodeficiency virus (HIV) or symptoms suggestive of TB (**Fig. 3**). In addition, children aged 2 to 14 years examined in countries with TB incidence of 20 per 100,000 or higher receive a tuberculin skin test (TST, 2007–2018) or interferon gamma release assay (IGRA, 2009–present) test; if positive, a chest radiograph is required. Applicants diagnosed with active TB must complete treatment by direct observed therapy before they are cleared to travel to the United States. Implementation initially focused on high-volume countries with high TB rates, with the goal of global implementation among more than 600 Panel Physicians in 159 countries (**Fig. 4**).

Regional Panel Physician trainings, involving panel staff from 127 countries between 2008 and 2016 (and counting), have been key in disseminating the 2007 TBTI guidelines. In each country, DGMQ/CDC works to link Panel Physician programs with broader national TB control efforts. Data suggest that US investment in TB control programs within source countries yields greater returns on investment than improvement of screening algorithms alone,[14] and TBTI implementation efforts have included laboratory capacity building, expanding many laboratories with the ability to perform TB cultures in implementing countries. Some laboratories also developed the capacity to test for resistance to second-line TB drugs, and hence to identify cases of multidrug-resistant (MDR) TB.[15]

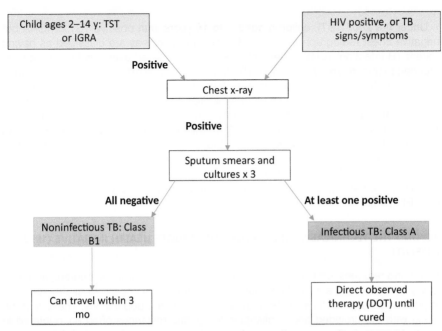

Fig. 3. 2007 TBTI: culture and directly observed therapy. (*Courtesy of* DGMQ/CDC.)

A 2015 analysis found that after 2007 TBTI implementation, overseas TB detection rates in US-bound immigrants and refugees increased by >600 cases per year. In turn, the annual number of reported cases in foreign-born individuals within a year after arrival in the United States, which had previously been relatively constant, declined from 1511 cases in 2007 to 940 cases in 2012.[16]

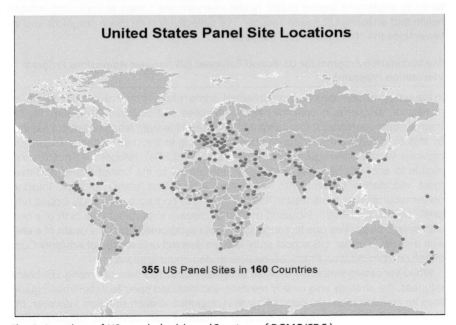

Fig. 4. Locations of US panel physicians. (*Courtesy of* DGMQ/CDC.)

Under the 2007 TBTI, children aged 2 to 14 years with positive TST or IGRA but negative chest radiograph or other TB evaluation overseas are classified as having "latent TB infection" (LTBI). These children are not treated overseas but are recommended to undergo reevaluation for TB after arrival.[17] A 2010 assessment determined that only 70% of immigrant and refugee children classified with LTBI overseas (themselves constituting 12% of all children evaluated overseas) received the recommended postarrival evaluation; of those confirmed to have LTBI, only 30% completed the full course of therapy. Further, 71% of children diagnosed with LTBI overseas by TST had a negative IGRA after arrival in the United States.[18] IGRA-based TB testing represents a new frontier for our program, and has replaced TST in the latest update to the TBTIs (2017).[17] Use of IGRA may limit overdiagnosis of LTBI in a population screened overseas, and help improve rates of postarrival evaluation and completion of LTBI therapy.

BEYOND THE TECHNICAL INSTRUCTIONS: THE REFUGEE HEALTH INITIATIVE (1999–PRESENT)

US-bound refugees live in diverse settings, including camps, urban centers, and rural areas, in their home and asylum countries. Limitations in access to health services, imposed by war and displacement, affect many refugee populations. These factors, along with the crowded and challenging living circumstances often encountered in refugee camps or other temporary asylum settings, expose refugees to infectious disease outbreaks and other health conditions. DGMQ/CDC has partnered with camp-based and other international refugee health agencies to investigate and mitigate disease outbreaks and build laboratory capacity.

Whereas immigrants travel to the United States individually or with their families, refugees resettle in groups, on a predetermined schedule, with a 3-month to 6-month window between medical examination and departure. This window affords an opportunity to implement limited public health interventions aimed at improving refugee health and ensuring US health security. We collectively term these programs and interventions the "Refugee Health Initiative."

The Vaccination Program for US-Bound Refugees (US Refugee Admissions Program Vaccination Program)

In the setting of displacement and upheaval, some refugees may be excluded from immunization programs in both their home countries and countries of asylum, leaving them susceptible to vaccine-preventable diseases. However, refugees are not required by statute to receive immunizations before traveling to the United States. The statute provides vaccination requirements for immigrants (LPRs); refugees do not become eligible to apply to be LPRs until 1 year after arrival to the United States and must meet vaccination requirements when they adjust their status to LPR. Vaccine-preventable disease transmission has led to serious consequences in US-bound refugees, especially children, including morbidity, disease importation, the birth of a child with severe disabilities due to congenital rubella syndrome,[19] and the death of a child with measles. Further, US school entry is often delayed until receipt of Advisory Committee on Immunization Practices–recommended immunizations.

When vaccine-preventable disease outbreaks occurred near or among US-bound refugees, the strategy was initially reactive, and included specific, time-limited guidelines for immunization and delay of travel in response to each situation. However, this strategy delayed immunization until after outbreaks were detected, resulting in imported cases, did nothing to prevent future outbreaks, and was very costly. For example, international and domestic costs for just one of these outbreaks were estimated at $130,000, partly due to the high costs of travel cancellations and rebookings.[20]

Following these and other experiences, DGMQ/CDC developed a routine immunization schedule for US-bound refugees, in close consultation with CDC vaccine-preventable disease experts. The resulting Vaccination Program for US-bound Refugees is cofunded by DGMQ/CDC and the US Department of State, which funds the overseas medical examination of US-bound refugees; the International Organization for Migration (IOM) is the main implementing partner overseas. Starting in 2 countries, this vaccination program has expanded to nearly 60, more than three-quarters of program sites, with a goal of reaching all sites within the next year. The program is based on US standards, and includes specific guidelines for cold chain maintenance, monitoring, documentation, and adverse events reporting. The program's immunization schedule now includes 11 vaccines, protecting against 14 diseases (**Box 1**).

Although immunization still is not required for resettlement, it is highly recommended to US-bound refugees, for the important health benefits and protection conferred to refugees and their receiving communities, and to prevent travel delays. Most US-bound refugees have opted in, with more than 260,000 benefiting from the Vaccination Program since 2012. In FY 2018, approximately 90% of arriving refugees received at least 1 age-appropriate dose of measles vaccine, according to DGMQ/CDC EDN data. Further, whereas in prior years many vaccine-preventable disease outbreaks (measles, mumps, polio, varicella, influenza, meningococcemia, and others) resulted in morbidity and costly travel delays, since FY 2016, the year with the largest number of resettling refugees since 1995, there have been no group travel delays associated with vaccine-preventable diseases, as of the time of writing. Net cost savings related to the USRAP Vaccination Program have been estimated at $225 per person.[21]

Box 1
Components of immunization schedule for US-bound refugees, fiscal year 2018[a]

Diphtheria, tetanus, and pertussis (DTP or DTaP) vaccine

Hepatitis B vaccine

H influenzae type b (Hib) vaccine[b]

Measles, mumps, and rubella (MMR) vaccine[c]

Oral polio vaccine (OPV)[c] or inactivated polio vaccine (IPV)

Pneumococcal vaccine[b]

Rotavirus vaccine[c]

Tetanus and diphtheria (Td) vaccine

Meningococcal ACWY vaccine[b]

Varicella vaccine[c]

Influenza vaccine (selected sites only)

[a] Up to 2 doses of each vaccine, depending on age and availability.

[b] Additional doses or separate recommendations may apply for patients with certain medical conditions.

[c] Vaccines contraindicated in immunocompromised or pregnant patients.

Courtesy of DGMQ/CDC.

Presumptive Treatment for Parasitic Infections

Displacement combined with crowded, difficult living conditions also leaves refugees exposed to parasitic diseases and other neglected tropical diseases. For example, a 1997 assessment of US-bound Barawan Somali refugees showed that 7% had malaria and 38% had intestinal parasites[22]; in a 2004 assessment of resettled Lost Boys and Girls from Sudan, 44% were *Schistosoma*-seropositive and 46% *Strongyloides*-seropositive.[23] Based on this and other evidence, DGMQ/CDC developed a presumptive parasite treatment schedule for US-bound refugees, including 2 to 4 drugs targeting intestinal helminths, *Strongyloides stercoralis*, *Schistosoma* spp, and *Plasmodium falciparum*, at overseas departure based on country of origin and examination (**Table 1**).

This mass drug treatment[24] initiative has significantly reduced the burden of parasitic diseases in US-bound refugees. For example, a 1999 evaluation comparing refugees arriving in Minnesota before and after the presumptive treatment intervention (n = 27,000) showed a significant decline in stool helminth prevalence, from 22.5% to 7.5%, after a single dose of albendazole was instituted just before overseas departure.[25] A longitudinal evaluation of US-bound refugees conducted between 2012 and 2015 showed similar declines in intestinal helminths by stool polymerase chain reaction (PCR), and, for the first time, demonstrated declines in *Strongyloides* prevalence both by stool PCR and serologic assays after presumptive treatment with ivermectin.[26] Finally, an evaluation conducted in Minnesota showed essential elimination of malaria occurring after resettlement in arriving West African refugees after a single predeparture dose of sulfadoxine-pyrimethamine. The medication has since been changed to Coartem (artemether/lumefantrine) because of regional resistance.[27]

Predeparture mass drug administration programs for parasitic infections confer both health and cost benefits. A 2016 analysis estimated that although both approaches would reduce parasite burden at similar rates, it is approximately sixfold less expensive to treat presumptively before departure than to screen and treat refugees after arrival.[28]

Table 1
Centers for Disease Control and Prevention recommendations for overseas presumptive parasite treatment in US-bound refugees

Region	Coartem (Malaria)	Praziquantel (Schistosomiasis)	Albendazole (Soil-Transmitted Helminths)	Ivermectin (Strongyloides)
Africa, non-Loa Loa areas	√	√	√	Burundi, Ethiopia, Kenya, Rwanda, Uganda, Tanzania
Africa, Loa Loa areas	√	√	√	Not recommended
Asia	Not recommended	Not recommended	√	Nepal, Malaysia, Thailand
Middle East	Not recommended	Not recommended	√	Jordan, Iraq, Egypt
Latin America	Not recommended	Not recommended	√	Future consideration

Courtesy of DGMQ/CDC.

Fitness to Fly: Predeparture Medical Screening

Some refugees may have other medical conditions that do not pose a public health risk, but may affect their health during travel, and must be managed before or during travel or immediately after arrival. Conditions resulting in severe illness or death in US-bound refugees during transit have included congenital cardiac disease, sickle cell disease, and malnutrition, among others.

DGMQ/CDC collaborates closely with partners such as IOM to develop and implement screening protocols to identify, manage, and stabilize patients with these and other chronic medical conditions before departure, with the goal of improving travel fitness. These protocols ensure that necessary referrals are completed and medications are refilled, that patients in need of specific interventions before travel (eg, blood transfusions for patients with hemoglobinopathies) receive them, and that the medical staff and equipment needed to facilitate a safe and comfortable flight are secured.

Site-Specific Clinical Protocols

Some clinical standard operating procedures were developed with specific populations in mind. For example, in 2014 IOM and states notified DGMQ/CDC of cases of splenomegaly, affecting approximately 15% of refugees resettling from Uganda. Contributing factors may include malaria, schistosomiasis, malnutrition, hepatitis, or hematologic conditions.[29] Because appropriate pretravel management may reduce the risk of splenic rupture and other complications, evaluation and management protocols were developed, detailing important history and physical examination items, workup considerations (eg, ultrasound and testing for malaria, hepatitis, sickle cell, and anemia), and travel preparation measures.

GUIDELINES FOR THE DOMESTIC MEDICAL EXAMINATION: PROMOTING REFUGEE HEALTH AFTER ARRIVAL

In addition to the overseas activities described, DGMQ/CDC recommends a more comprehensive medical evaluation after arrival in the United States. Facilitated by state public health departments, state Refugee Health Coordinators, and other partners, this examination is not required for the resettlement process but is intended to identify health concerns and minimize morbidity. It is typically conducted 1 to 3 months after arrival. DGMQ/CDC developed evidence-based guidelines and checklists to help receiving states perform this evaluation. Items covered include the history and physical examination; screening for hepatitis and HIV infection; domestic immunization guidelines; and guidance for assessment of nutritional status and testing for elevated blood lead levels, sexually transmitted diseases (STDs), TB, malaria, and intestinal parasites.[30] Immunization catch-up is typically initiated during this examination, although not all sites are able to follow patients longitudinally to completion of the full immunization series.

To further assist state health partners in identifying common health conditions in diverse US-bound populations, DGMQ/CDC has compiled health profiles, describing population background, routes of movement and asylum, and priority health conditions for the largest arriving refugee groups. These profiles are updated over time to reflect newer arriving populations.[31]

SUMMARY

Forced displacement and migration have increased to record levels in today's geopolitical environment; hence, ensuring both the health of migrating populations and the health security of receiving countries is of critical importance. Based on 22 years of experience in developing and monitoring a health assessment framework for US-bound immigrants and refugees, DGMQ/CDC has identified successful strategies to improve health during planned migrations. These overseas screening, treatment, and vaccination initiatives have reduced US TB rates; decreased transmission and importation of vaccine-preventable diseases; prevented morbidity from parasitic diseases; and saved domestic health costs. Beyond their importance in the planned migration setting, these initiatives may offer a valuable template that can be adapted during unplanned migrations. For example, efforts to anticipate the flow of asylum seekers over the full course of their journey, from origin to destination, could allow for preventive and curative interventions that would improve health security. Such public health interventions can be perceived as triple-wins: good for migrants, good for sending communities, and good for receiving communities.

ACKNOWLEDGMENTS

The authors thank Zanju Wang and Courtney Chappelle of CDC's Immigrant, Refugee, and Migrant Health Branch, Division of Global Migration and Quarantine, for their contributions to data mapping.

REFERENCES

1. Murphy FA, Nathanson N. The emergence of new virus diseases: an overview. Sem Virol 1994;5:87–102.
2. United Nations. Refugees and migrants: definitions. Available at: https://refugeesmigrants.un.org/definitions. Accessed September 21, 2018.
3. UNHCR. Figures at a glance. Available at: http://www.unhcr.org/figures-at-a-glance.html. Accessed September 21, 2018.
4. US Department of Homeland Security. Refugees and asylees. 2018. Available at: https://www.dhs.gov/immigration-statistics/refugees-asylees. Accessed September 21, 2018.
5. The World Bank. Refugee population by country or territory of asylum. In: Data. 2018. Available at: https://data.worldbank.org/indicator/SM.POP.REFG?year_high_desc=true. Accessed September 21, 2018.
6. UNHCR. Resettlement. 2018. Available at: http://www.unhcr.org/resettlement.html. Accessed September 21, 2018.
7. US Department of State US Refugee Admissions Program. 2018. Available at: https://www.state.gov/j/prm/ra/admissions/index.htm. Accessed September 21, 2018.
8. Refugee Processing Center. Admissions & arrivals. Available at: http://www.wrapsnet.org/admissions-and-arrivals/. Accessed September 21, 2018.
9. US Department of Homeland Security. Immigration statistics. Available at: https://www.dhs.gov/immigration-statistics. Accessed September 21, 2018.
10. Centers for Disease Control and Prevention. Medical examination of immigrants and refugees. Available at: https://www.cdc.gov/immigrantrefugeehealth/exams/medical-examination.html. Accessed September 21, 2018.
11. Centers for Disease Control and Prevention. Reported tuberculosis in the United States, . Tuberculosis, data and statistics. Available at: https://www.cdc.gov/tb/statistics/reports/2016/default.htm. Accessed September 21, 2018.
12. Maloney S, Fielding K, Laserson K, et al. Assessing the performance of overseas tuberculosis screening programs. Arch Intern Med 2006;166:234–40.

13. Liu Y, Weinberg MS, Ortega LS, et al. Overseas screening for tuberculosis in US-bound immigrants and refugees. N Engl J Med 2009;360(23):2406–15.
14. Schwartzman K, Oxlade O, Barr G, et al. Domestic returns from investment in the control of tuberculosis in other countries. N Engl J Med 2005;353(10):1008–20.
15. Douglas P, Posey DL, Zenner D, et al. Capacity strengthening through pre-migration tuberculosis screening programmes: IRHWG experiences. Int J Tuberc Lung Dis 2017;21(7):737–45.
16. Liu Y, Posey D, Cetron M, et al. Effect of a culture-based screening algorithm on tuberculosis incidence in immigrants and refugees bound for the United States. Ann Intern Med 2015;162(6):420–8.
17. Centers for Disease Control and Prevention. Tuberculosis technical instructions for panel physicians. Available at: https://www.cdc.gov/immigrantrefugeehealth/exams/ti/panel/tuberculosis-panel-technical-instructions.html. Accessed September 21 and November 19, 2018.
18. Taylor EM, Painter J, Posey D, et al. Latent tuberculosis infection among immigrant and refugee children in the United States: 2010. J Immigr Minor Health 2016;18(5):966–70.
19. Centers for Disease Control and Prevention. Brief report: Imported case of congenital rubella syndrome–New Hampshire, 2005. MMWR Morb Mortal Wkly Rep 2005;54(45):1160–1.
20. Coleman MS, Burke HM, Welstead BL, et al. Cost analysis of measles in refugees arriving at Los Angeles International Airport from Malaysia. Hum Vaccin Immunother 2017;13(5):1084–90.
21. Joo H, Maskery B, Joo H, et al. A comparative cost analysis of the Vaccination Program for US-bound Refugees. Vaccine 2018;36(20):2896–901.
22. Centers for Disease Control and Prevention. Domestic intestinal parasite guidelines. Available at: https://www.cdc.gov/immigrantrefugeehealth/guidelines/domestic/intestinal-parasites-domestic.html. Accessed September 21, 2018.
23. Posey DL, Blackburn BG, Weinberg M, et al. High prevalence and presumptive treatment of schistosomiasis and strongyloidiasis among African refugees. Clin Infect Dis 2007;45(10):1310–5.
24. World Health Organization. Preventive therapy in human helminthiasis. Geneva (United Kingdom): World Health Organization; 2006.
25. Swanson S, Phares CR, Mamo B, et al. Albendazole therapy and enteric parasites in United States-bound refugees. N Engl J Med 2012;366(16):1498–507.
26. Mitchell T, Lee D, Weinberg M, et al. Impact of enhanced health interventions for United States-bound refugees: evaluating best practices in migration health. Am J Trop Med Hyg 2018;98(3):920–8.
27. Collinet-Adler S, Stauffer WM, Boulware DR, et al. Financial implications of refugee malaria: the impact of pre-departure presumptive treatment with anti-malarial drugs. Am J Trop Med Hyg 2007;77(3):458–63.
28. Maskery B, Coleman MS, Weinberg M, et al. Economic analysis of the impact of overseas and domestic treatment and screening options for intestinal helminth infection among US-Bound Refugees from Asia. PLoS Negl Trop Dis 2016;10(8):e0004910.
29. Goers M, Ope M, Samuels A, et al. Notes from the field: splenomegaly of unknown etiology in Congolese refugees applying for resettlement to the United States—Uganda, 2015. MMWR Morb Mortal Wkly Rep 2016;65(35):943–4.

30. Centers for Disease Control and Prevention. Guidelines for the US domestic medical examination for newly arriving refugees. Available at: https://www.cdc.gov/immigrantrefugeehealth/guidelines/domestic/domestic-guidelines.html. Accessed September 21, 2018..

31. Centers for Disease Control and Prevention. Refugee health profiles. Available at: https://www.cdc.gov/immigrantrefugeehealth/profiles/index.html. Accessed September 21, 2018..

The Intersection of Urban and Global Health

Nora L. Jones, PhD[a],*, Julia Burger, MD, MA[b], Ashleigh Hall, DO, MA[b],
Kathleen A. Reeves, MD[a]

KEYWORDS

- Urban health • Global health • Health inequity • Social determinants of health
- Health disparities

KEY POINTS

- Global health and urban health are more related than often understood.
- Health care in underserved urban areas can benefit from the same attention to engagement found in global health professionalism.
- Sustainable and successful health care interventions require community engagement.
- The provision of health in underserved areas needs to pay more attention to the social, political, economic, and other cultural forces impacting the communities served.

INTRODUCTION

Health is most commonly defined as "a state of complete physical, mental and social well-being and not merely the absence of disease or infirmity."[1] That this definition has persisted, unamended, since its initial adoption by the World Health Organization in 1948[2] illustrates the strength of this understanding. Although this foundational definition of health remains unchanged, academic medicine has broken down the broader definition into specialized foci, such as rural, urban, global, international, academic, and community-based health. One of the reasons for this differentiation is to direct training that better serves a more well-defined population. It also, however, has led to territory marking and conflict over medical education and the practice of health care. What follows is an exploration of the opportunities for pediatricians to think, practice, and teach at the intersection of two of these fields: global and urban health. Although not commonly thought of as similar in the professional community or in the literature in general, each can learn much from the other to further patient center the care provided. The concepts we put forward in this Introduction are summarized in **Fig. 1.**

[a] Center for Bioethics, Urban Health, and Policy, Lewis Katz School of Medicine at Temple University, 3500 North Broad Street, Suite 324, Philadelphia, PA 19140, USA; [b] Department of Pediatrics, Lewis Katz School of Medicine at Temple University, 3223 North Broad Street, 1st Floor, Old Dental School, Philadelphia, PA 19140, USA
* Corresponding author.
E-mail address: nora.jones@temple.edu

Pediatr Clin N Am 66 (2019) 561–573
https://doi.org/10.1016/j.pcl.2019.02.005
0031-3955/19/© 2019 Elsevier Inc. All rights reserved.

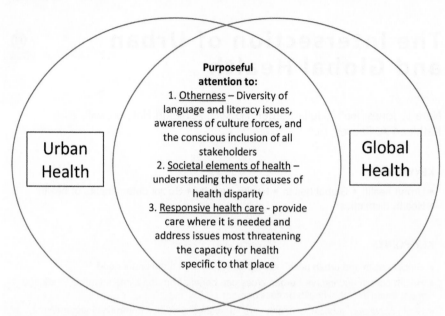

Fig. 1. The intersection of urban and global health.

Global health "feels" different from many of the other foci because it involves pro-viders intentionally traveling to a foreign location and working with people who are usually very different from themselves in terms of general demographics and world-view. Global health can be very focused on the "other," a generic term used to describe people not only from a different place, but with different experiences and worldviews. Global health's conscious awareness of this otherness is reflected in its educational competencies, including attention to language and literacy issues, aware-ness of culture forces, and the conscious inclusion of all stakeholders in deciding how, when, and where to provide care.[3,4] Such purposeful attention to the diversity of the other is central to professionalism within global health.

Urban health has not carried that same sense of other. Disparities that exist in urban communities have historically been seen to result from factors related to personal accountability, and a common proposed remedy includes highlighting the need for behavioral change, accomplished with education.[5] More recently, there has been an understanding of the role of social determinants on health and on the impact on health of societal ills like poverty, food insecurity, poor educational systems, and transporta-tion issues.[6,7] Despite their importance, these factors are too often considered to be out of the purview of the health care provider, and thus not factored into the structure or practice of health care. In addition, much less emphasis is placed on a sense of other, even though the people providing the care in urban distressed communities are rarely from the communities they are serving. Urban health care is not generally provided in a way that responds to what the community needs or how the community would best be able to take advantage of the services. Health care in urban, distressed communities is delivered, just as all other health care in the United States is delivered: it is centered around the providers and is more often reactive to disease rather than directed at providing opportunities for health.

Perhaps the biggest difference between global health and urban health practitioners is in how each understands the root causes of health disparities. It is our observation, stemming from a collective of more than 50 years of experience in urban academic medical centers, that providers, as well as the other stakeholders in a health care system, approach the disparities within our urban underserved populations as having their root causes in the beliefs, attitudes, and behaviors of our patients themselves. Such an approach is in many ways distinctly American, given that the United States is a country whose identity is rooted in an ideology of equality and equal opportunity. Under such a worldview, individuals who are less well off, less healthy, or less educated are so because they have failed to pull themselves up by their bootstraps. Global health practitioners, in contrast, do not generally think of the particular patients they see as being responsible for their need for health care. Fault for poor health is found in political, economic, and other social forces and policies that disproportionately and negatively impact vulnerable populations. We present the argument that understanding social determinants and their history as a primary causal mechanism is a skill from the global health toolbox that those of us working in urban health need to embrace. If we can better understand the factors that lead to unquestioned and uncritical acceptance of medical need of patients in global settings, we can perhaps replicate those factors and, thus, be better positioned to achieve similar successes.

A second major difference between global and urban health is seen in how each field approaches their respective populations. Urban health care institutions rarely define the population they serve as the community surrounding the health system, which is perhaps why residents of communities in the shadows of urban academic medical centers are often the least healthy individuals within a city. It is our contention that one of the main reasons this disparity exists is due to the secondary safety net systems that urban health centers create to serve the urban distressed community. A safety net system is not tailorable to any particular community, but is more of a minimal public health requirement. Following a different approach, global health practitioners provide care where it is needed and address the issues most threatening the capacity for health specific to that place. Such an approach could mean addressing communicable diseases and vaccination, facilitating clean drinking water, aiding access to sustainable nutrition, or fostering the ability to provide long-term access to medications. Global health provides health care specific to the needs of the community they are serving and does not have a safety net mentality for the communities they serve.

We are arguing that there is a usefulness to exploring the intersection between global and urban health, and that global and urban practitioners and educators can learn from each other to provide better, more focused care in each specific setting. To illustrate this point, we focus on 2 specific guiding principles within global health—otherness and engagement—that, if applied to the provision of urban health, would greatly improve health equity in urban distressed communities. We discuss 3 specific innovative interventions that apply these principles and reflect this promise. Finally, we review the current movement within academic medical centers in the United States to concentrate on urban health–related curricula and how that impetus can help to inform a more sustained approach to effective and comprehensive global health programs throughout the world.

REFINING THE DEFINITION OF URBAN HEALTH

Before continuing, we need to clarify what exactly we are referring to when we use the term urban health. The term refers, at its most basic level, to health in urban spaces. It is often contrasted with rural health, and refers to the provision of health care in areas that are dense and diverse, with economic, health, and other social disparities. Although not often overtly stated, urban health does not apply to all populations within urban centers. Residents of wealthier urban neighborhoods with comprehensive private insurance and accessible high-quality health care do not merit particular concern in medicine because these individuals do not lack access, insurance, or other resources related to health; in other words, they have the capacity to be healthy.

The lack of full capacity to be healthy is more prevalent in urban communities with fewer socioeconomic, educational, and financial resources, with limited access to healthy foods and safe streets, and with less political and social power. Such social determinants are critical for the capacity to be healthy because social and economic forces are overwhelmingly responsible for any individual's overall morbidity and mortality[8] **(Fig. 2)**. A life expectancy project sponsored by the National Center for Health Statistics and the Robert Wood Johnson Foundation starkly illustrated the correlation of life expectancy with zip code.[9] Our city, Philadelphia, has the distinction of being the city with the second greatest life expectancy disparity in the United States; residents of neighborhoods separated by 4.4 miles experience a 20-year disparity in life expectancy.

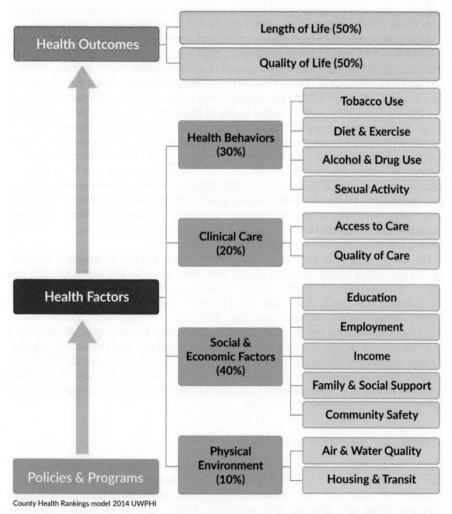

County Health Rankings model 2014 UWPHI

Fig. 2. County health rankings model. (*Courtesy of* University of Wisconsin-Madison Population Health Institute.)

The repeated examples of such extreme disparities over small geographic areas supports the argument that geographic location is a stronger predictor of health than race, gender, educational attainment, insurance status, or any other demographic variable alone. Geographic location is, however, complexly intertwined with these other demographics, and the variables cannot be so easily disentangled in life as they can in epidemiologic statistics. What this means is that people of color, poor people, and otherwise marginalized individuals in the United States are living in circumstances as disparate and distinct from each other as the United States is to developing countries. As inequities in the United States continue to increase, the phrase "the local is global" takes on new implications, and it is to these that we now turn.

Otherness

The health care workforce in the United States does not generally reflect the people who live in our urban, distressed communities. Very few practitioners live in the neighborhoods that surround our urban academic medical centers, making it more likely that they know relatively little about the history, context, strengths, and challenges of the communities where their patients live. Seeing community members only in the clinic, in moments of need, pain, and powerlessness, can result in significant bias, poor communication, a lack of trust, and an eventual lack of empathy. In stark contrast, before global health practitioners embark on a project, there is an expectation that they learn the history, strengths, challenges, culture, and context of the community to which they are traveling.[10] This process allows for a greater sense of empathy, better communication, more trust, less marginalization, and less bias.

In 2012, our center created a master of arts degree in urban bioethics (www.temple.edu/bioethics) with the explicit purpose of looking at disparities in health as not only inequitable, but as unethical. We also wanted current and future health care providers (as well as researchers, administrators, and others) who are not knowledgeable about the urban community in which they find themselves, to gain a methodologic toolbox to become informed and be aware of otherness. Thus, students spend the second year of the program embedded into the community to learn from and work with community members. The goal of this course is to learn how to do this in any urban, distressed setting. Our graduates have shared with us how this experience has changed their practice of medicine, relieving some of their moral distress and better working with patients to successfully foster health. In light of this success, we have started a less intense, but longitudinal and mandatory, service learning program for all medical students. We are in the process of evaluating whether this experience changes their attitudes toward and understanding of urban communities as well as their ability to maintain empathy throughout their practice.

Engagement

Hospitals in rural America, suburban America, and urban America look and function very similarly. However, the issues impacting health in these distinct areas differ dramatically. Global health concentrates on a specific geographic area and focuses on what is most affecting that particular area, whether it be an infectious epidemic, a resource problem like clean water, a policy impacting health, an educational need for providers, or many other possible scenarios. They then direct the work and care delivery to the most pressing needs of that particular place.[11,12] Our center has taken this lesson and applied it to the communities in the shadows of our academic medical center. Our first example illustrates a success story that began by listening to community voices, and the second focuses on an educational program founded on this principle.

Philadelphia CeaseFire

In 2010, our center completed a needs assessment of our urban catchment area that included a number of focus groups with influential and connected community members to learn what this community felt were the most pressing issues for them regarding health. Instead of diabetes, cardiovascular disease, and obesity, 3 clinical conditions whose prevalence is most starkly evident in epidemiologic studies of the area, violence was the most concerning problem for the majority of the residents, followed closely by the related issue of opportunities for their children. It is our contention that our ability to see these nonclinical factors as major health issues in the same way as global health providers see epidemics and clean water as central to providing health is imperative if urban centers are ever to positively address health disparities. Therefore, as a result of this information, we created a violence prevention model based on the premise supported by the Centers for Disease Control and Prevention that violence is a public health epidemic.[13] This program, Philadelphia CeaseFire (www.philaceasefire.com), hires ex offenders and trains them in conflict mediation so they can serve as credible messengers in their own communities, acting much like Centers for Disease Control and Prevention workers do in an epidemic: intervene when violence is happening, mediate people away from violence toward opportunity, and "vaccinate" high-risk individuals with education and employment. The model is based on Cure Violence, a program developed by an infectious disease physician, Dr Gary Slutkin.[14] In the last 2 years, our results show a 30% decrease in violence in areas of the city that had CeaseFire teams versus areas that had similar rates of violence and did not have CeaseFire teams. If implemented throughout our urban distressed community, this would result in 400 fewer shootings per year. Very little improves access to health than not being a victim of violence.

The Pincus Urban Health Fellowship

To help health care providers in urban settings be better prepared to respond to the needs of urban communities, we partnered with a local philanthropic organization to create the Pincus Family Foundation Pediatric Urban Health Fellowship. This program is directed toward junior clinicians interested in learning the skills needed to create, fund, and implement innovative programs based on community engagement principles that will work to improve the overall health of children in urban, distressed communities. We graduated our first fellows in 2018. Their research, presented herein, reflects many of the themes we are discussing.

The role of trauma-informed care in urban communities The origin and evolution of attention to Adverse Childhood Experience (ACE) is an example of how an engaged approach to addressing an "epidemic" more evident in urban distressed communities can yield incredible insight. ACEs were first defined in the late 1990s by Felitti and associates[15] based on their survey of middle class adult patients in the Kaiser Permanente Health System in Southern California that correlated different types of stressful experiences in childhood with chronic disease and health outcomes later in life. With 2 waves of survey data covering more than 17,000 adults, these original ACE studies found that two-thirds of participants had exposure to at least 1 ACE, and 1 in 9 had an ACE score of 5 or more.[16] In addition to revealing that ACEs were more common than many had expected, the study found a graded relationship between number of ACEs and adult risk behaviors and diseases[15,16] (**Fig. 3**).

The import of these powerful results has limited generalizability in 2 respects, however. Demographically, the original ACEs studies surveyed primarily white, upper middle class, college educated, and insured individuals. Individuals living and

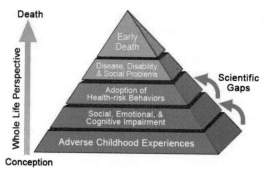

Fig. 3. Adverse childhood experiences pyramid. (*From* Substance Abuse and Mental Health Services Administration. Adverse Childhood Experiences. Available at: https://www.samhsa.gov/capt/practicing-effective-prevention/prevention-behavioral-health/adverse-childhood-experiences. Accessed January 31, 2019.)

working in more diverse urban environments also found that the ACEs from the original study did not address their neighborhood and community experiences that created significant sources of stress. This concern led to the development of the Urban ACE study in Philadelphia.[17] Through literature review as well as qualitative data from African American and Latino youth in Philadelphia, the themes of the expanded ACEs were developed to include factors related to social location, such as exposure to community violence, experiencing racism, living in an unsafe neighborhood, experiencing bullying, and having a history of living in foster care (**Fig. 4**). The results of the Urban ACE study showed that the prevalence of the conventional ACEs was higher in the Philadelphia dataset compared with the original and most other subsequent

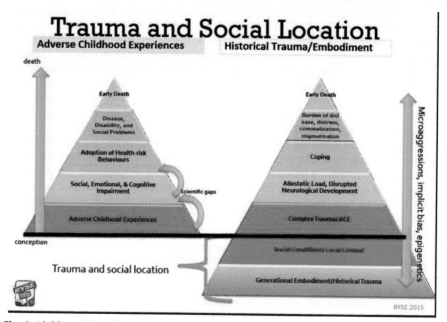

Fig. 4. Linking ACEs with social location and historical trauma. (*From* RYSE Center. Available at: https://www.acesconnection.com/blog/adding-layers-to-the-aces-pyramid-what-do-you-think. Accessed January 31, 2019.)

studies: 72.9% of Philadelphians had at least 1 conventional ACE, 47.6% had 1 to 3 ACEs, and 20.7% were found to have an ACE score of 4 or more. For the 5 Expanded ACEs, they found that 63.4% of the population surveyed had at least 1 exposure, 50% had a score of 1 to 3 ACEs, and 13.4% had 3 or more. A further analysis of the expanded ACEs found that 40.5% of participants had witnessed community violence, 34.5% experienced racial discrimination, and 27.3% felt their neighborhood was unsafe. The most distressed, urban neighborhoods in Philadelphia are in north Philadelphia, surrounding our health system, and ACE surveys from these communities reported that more than 48% of adults experienced 4 or more adverse childhood experiences.

Despite the scope of research on the impact of toxic stress, there remain children who succeed despite difficult circumstances. Resilience, or the ability to cope or adapt in response to risk, adversity, or challenge, has come to be the most commonly understood factor for such success. It is not inherent or unique to certain individuals, but is a dynamic concept that builds on individual strengths rather than emphasizing deficits. Resilience develops over time and can be fostered.[18] Many investigators make the assumption that greater resilience can mitigate the detrimental effects of ACEs; however, the correlation of resilience scores with long-term health outcomes is largely unknown. Two adult studies and 2 pediatric studies, all published in Europe, seem to show better health outcomes with higher measures of resilience,[19–22] but the question of whether resilience can mitigate the health effects of ACEs remains unexplored. Based on this existing knowledge and the current knowledge gap, we developed a research study, currently in the data collection phase, to examine the relation between resilience scores, ACE scores, and health outcomes in adolescents, particularly blood pressure, body mass index, and depression.

The results of this study can help us to direct where to focus intervention programs. If greater resilience is found to be associated with better health outcomes, then building resilience is a beneficial intervention to pursue. Additionally, with the resilience tool being used in this study we can further break down the resilience score into subscales looking more in depth at personal contributors, family contributors, and community contributors to resilience. This process can also help further refine where to target interventions. The data suggest that, for an urban health center to become engaged in addressing the most pressing issues of that community, the health center must become a trauma-informed institution. Data from decade long studies funded by the Robert Wood Johnson Foundation found that trauma-informed practices had a statistically significant positive impact on a community's overall health.[23] A trauma-informed approach is defined by the Substance Abuse and Mental Health Services Association as "a program or organization that 1. *Realizes* the widespread impact of trauma and understands potential paths for recovery; 2. *Recognizes* the signs and symptoms of trauma in clients, families, staff, and others involved with the system; 3. *Responds* by fully integrating knowledge about trauma into policies, procedures, and practices; and 4. Seeks to actively resist *re-traumatization.*"[24] Beyond the clinic or health system culture shift, work can continue to be done at the policy level creating more just systems that fight inequity in resources, access to schools, housing, and health care, therefore preventing some ACEs from occurring in the first place. We will also benefit from more engaged collaboration with schools, community programs, and places of worship, among others, to create a safety net for children and their families to help them nurture, grow, protect, and heal. We should strive for a more just, equitable society. That goal means addressing the inequities associated with ACEs now, and also addressing ACEs, offering healing, and resilience building to prevent further inequities in the future.

Using a community-engaged app to promote health literacy Health literacy is a complicated concept at the intersection of health and education. It is defined by the Institute of Medicine as "the degree to which individuals have the capacity to obtain, process, and understand basic health information and services needed to make appropriate health decisions."[25] More recent definitions have begun to consider health literacy as an interaction between the demands of the health system and the skills of individuals, highlighting the skills of all parties involved in communication, providers included.[26]

Low health literacy is associated with limited health-related knowledge and comprehension, decreased mammography screening and influenza immunizations, increased emergency care visits and hospitalization rates, higher mortality rates, and increased health care expenditure.[27] Given the enormous costs of limited health literacy on economics and outcomes, it is not enough to simply address health literacy by changing our communication practices; we must also screen for health literacy levels and provide tailored education. When health literacy is thought of as a clinical problem, it essentially becomes a risk factor for poor outcomes. Therefore, we should screen for it in the same way we screen for other risk factors, like high blood pressure. We can also look at health literacy from a public health standpoint, considering health literacy as an asset that can be built on, like a diet that can be made healthier. Health literacy becomes "a means to enabling individuals to exert greater control over their health and the range of personal, social, and environmental determinants of health."[28] The public health model also starts with health literacy assessment, but the focus of the health care provider now shifts from only modifying communication to also helping patients to develop knowledge and skills in multiple areas that affect health. It allows for a broader range of interventions, including outside of the clinical setting. This process is very important, because only a very small portion of a person's health behaviors take place in the presence of a health care professional. In US health care today, it is often the emergency department that links individuals in their homes and communities with the health care institutions, and thus provides a potentially fruitful avenue for fostering health literacy.

In 2014, American children aged 17 years and younger made nearly 20 million visits to emergency department, which averages to nearly 54,800 visits per day.[29] It is estimated that between 58% and 82% of these visits were for nonurgent complaints, defined as one where the patient could "safely wait 2 to 3 hours or be seen by their regular doctor the next day."[30] Parents of children presenting to the pediatric emergency department (PED) for a nonurgent complaint are more likely than average to have a low health literacy level, slightly more than 50% per 1 year-long study of 1 urban PED,[31] compared with only 26% of parents nationally.[32] Low health literacy has been associated with a 50% increase in PED visits.[31]

One reason that parents may bring their children to the emergency department is that they overestimate the degree of illness.[33] If parents with low health literacy tend to overestimate their children's degree of illness and this leads to increased PED visits, then health literacy interventions, designed to enable individuals to exert greater control over their health, could be a potential intervention. Several studies have shown that educational interventions can be effective in fostering parents' confidence about their children's health and for eliminating unnecessary and costly PED visits.[34,35]

In an attempt to address overutilization of the emergency department, we have customized a pediatric symptom-checking smartphone app for our community. It supports decision making during acute illness, provides patient education, and is more convenient to use than a book or pamphlet. The content is owned by a company called Self Care Decisions (https://www.selfcare.info/) and is reviewed and updated at least yearly. Content is derived from the Schmitt -Thompson protocols, which are used by 90% of medical advice lines and more than 90% of pediatric practices nationally for triaging patients and providing advice. The symptom checking app offers the same advice on a mobile device platform and is written for caregivers on a sixth-grade level per the standards of the Centers for Medicare and Medicaid Services. It includes symptom care guides to help families make decisions about what level of care is needed (eg, emergency department vs pediatrician office) and it offers advice on both first aid and specific wellness and behavior topics. Our app uses the content described and has been customized for the North Philadelphia community. It lists resources such as breastfeeding support and local food banks. It also has a mapping feature to locate the nearest emergency department or urgent care center. In addition, 9-1-1 can be dialed directly through the app, as can a mental health crisis line. Our app allows clinicians to provide their patients with the tools they need to start making better health decisions. From an ethical standpoint, this supports a person's agency, or their capacity to act independently and make free choices. The more a person understands different options available to them, the better able they are to make a choice for themselves. Empowering people to make good choices can contribute to health equity. Meeting a person where they are on their own literacy level, and then providing them with appropriate educational materials in a way that encourages them to make the healthiest decisions possible could be one step toward overcoming health disparities. It is our hope that a symptom-checking smartphone app will prove to be a useful tool for achieving this goal. Data is being collected to understand how families use our app, and we expect to publish within the next two years.

SUMMARY

The most effective way to support the health of a community is to be sure that the community has access to a culturally appropriate, inclusive, well-educated health care workforce. Many medical schools and academic medical centers are beginning to focus their curricula around specific foci of health. Primary care tracks have a long history of success in training providers to be better prepared primary care physicians, especially in rural communities, and there are a number of programs dedicated to creating physician–scientists as well. Medical schools are increasingly looking at the value of urban and global health care tracks as well.

Although it is valuable for practitioners to be educated in a longitudinal global health experience before taking part in a global health program, it would be preferable for people from the community that needs service to be trained to provide that care, and global health programs are beginning to look at the importance of this educational model.[36] Urban health tracks are similarly working to build pipelines in urban communities that support and encourage young people through STEM education to successfully complete medical training. Such programs diversify the health care workforce so that more providers share context with more of the patients in urban, distressed communities. Urban programs need to help communities most in need around the world to develop more complete STEM programs as well as supportive, inclusive provider education that can help to build a workforce for every community across the globe that is more representative of that community.

No More Safety Net Hospitals

Historically, and before the rise of larger urban academic medical centers, health was directed to the community in which the providers reside, meaning that geography bound the provider with their patient population. Urban health centers see themselves

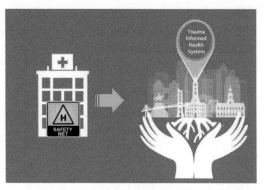

Fig. 5. From a safety net hospital to a trauma-informed health system.

at a disadvantage if they sit in an urban, distressed community because the majority of the people living in such areas receive medical assistance, and it is much more difficult for a health system to remain fiscally sustainable when a majority of their reimbursements are coming from Medicare and Medicaid. As a result, health systems structure themselves to attract a more lucrative patient, one with better insurance. Care provided to the local community becomes a secondary concern when strategic decisions are guided primarily by fiscal sustainability. The term safety net hospital is used to describe such institutions, and cities and institutions speak in ways demonstrating pride in being able to provide such needed safety net care. It is our contention that this is an unethical perspective to take. We should instead provide care to the direct community, fostering the capacity to be healthy with our strengths working in conjunction with whatever resources they have available (**Figs. 5** and **6**). We need to concentrate on the neighborhoods in our urban distressed communities and stop competing for the same, better insured patients. This effort will not only result in better health outcomes, but will also save significant amounts of money in health care expenditures. Such an approach fosters a holistic view of health both locally and globally.

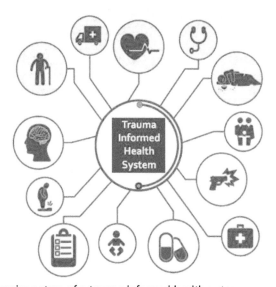

Fig. 6. Comprehensive nature of a trauma-informed health system.

ACKNOWLEDGMENTS

The authors thank Steuart Wright for his support in completing this article. Portions of the research and education initiatives discussed in this article were made possible through the support of and collaboration with the Pincus Family Foundation.

REFERENCES

1. World Health Organization. WHO Constitution. Available at: http://www.who.int/about/who-weare/constitution. Accessed March 13, 2019.
2. World Health Organization. WHO FAQ. Available at: http://www.who.int/suggestions/faq/en/. Accessed October 12, 2018.
3. Khan O, Guerrant R, Sanders J, et al. Global health education in US Medical schools. BMC Med Educ 2013;13(1):3–10.
4. Peluso M, Forrestel A, Hafler J, et al. Structured global health programs in US medical schools: a web-based review of certificates, tracks, and concentrations. Acad Med 2013;88(1):124–30.
5. Glanz K, Rimer BK, Viswanath K. Health behavior and health education: theory, research, and practice. Washington, DC: John Wiley & Sons; 2008.
6. Mullan F. Social mission in health professions education: beyond flexner. Jama 2017;318(2):122–3.
7. Smedley BD, Stith AY, Nelson AR. Unequal treatment. Confronting racial and ethnic disparities in health care, vol. 100. Washington, DC: The National Academy Press; 2003.
8. Remington PL, Catlin BB, Gennuso KP. The county health rankings: rationale and methods. Popul Health Metr 2015;13(1):11.
9. Arias E, Escobedo LA, Kennedy J, et al. US small-area life expectancy estimates project: methodology and results summary 2018. Available at: https://stacks.cdc.gov/view/cdc/58853.
10. Jogerst K, Callender B, Adams V, et al. Identifying interprofessional global health competencies for 21st-century health professionals. Ann Glob Health 2015;81(2):239–47.
11. Heck J, Pust R. A national consensus on the essential international-health curriculum for medical-schools. Acad Med 1993;68(8):596–8.
12. Battat R, Seidman G, Chadi N, et al. Global health competencies and approaches in medical education: a literature review. BMC Med Educ 2010;10(1):94–100.
13. Centers for Disease Control and Prevention. The history of violence as a public health issue 2016. Available at: https://www.cdc.gov/violenceprevention/pdf/history_violence-a.pdf. Accessed October 1, 2018.
14. Ransford C, Kane C, Slutkin G. Cure violence: a disease control approach to reduce violence and change behavior. In: Waltermaurer E, Akers TA, editors. Epidemiological criminology: theory to practice. Philadelphia: Taylor and Francis; 2013. p. 232–48.
15. Felitti V, Anda R, Nordenberg D, et al. Relationship of childhood abuse and household dysfunction to many of the leading causes of death in adults - The adverse childhood experiences (ACE) study. Am J Prev Med 1998;14(4):245–58.
16. Brown D, Anda R, Tiemeier H, et al. Adverse childhood experiences and the risk of premature mortality. Am J Prev Med 2009;37(5):389–96.
17. Cronholm P, Forke C, Wade R, et al. Adverse childhood experiences expanding the concept of adversity. Am J Prev Med 2015;49(3):354–61.
18. Harvard Center for the Developing Child. Available at: https://developingchild.harvard.edu/. Accessed July 16, 2018.

19. Crump C, Sundquist J, Winkleby M, et al. Low stress resilience in late adolescence and risk of hypertension in adulthood. Heart 2016;102(7):541–U576.
20. Hjemdal O, Aune T, Reinfjell T, et al. Resilience as a predictor of depressive symptoms: a correlational study with young adolescents. Clin Child Psychol Psychiatry 2007;12(1):91–104.
21. Stewart-Knox B, Duffy ME, Bunting B, et al. Associations between obesity (BMI and waist circumference) and socio-demographic factors, physical activity, dietary habits, life events, resilience, mood, perceived stress and hopelessness in healthy older Europeans. BMC public health 2012;12(1):424.
22. Schiel R, Kaps A, Stein G, et al. Identification of Predictors for Weight Reduction in Children and Adolescents with Overweight and Obesity (IDA-Insel Survey). Healthcare 2016;4(1):5.
23. Porter L, Martin K, Anda R. Self-healing communities: a transformational process model for improving intergenerational health. Princeton (NJ): Robert Wood Johnson Foundation; 2016.
24. Substance Abuse and Mental Health Services Administration. SAMHSA's concept of trauma and guidance for a trauma-informed approach. HHS Publication No. (SMA) 14-4884. Rockville (MD): Substance Abuse and Mental Health Services Administration; 2014.
25. Nielsen-Bohlman L, Panzer A, Kindig D, Institute of Medicine (US). Committee on Health Literacy. Health literacy: a prescription to end confusion. Washington, DC: National Academies Press; 2004.
26. Sørensen K, Van den Broucke S, Fullam J, et al. Health literacy and public health: a systematic review and integration of definitions and models. BMC public health 2012;12(1):80.
27. Berkman N, Sheridan S, Donahue K, et al. Low health literacy and health outcomes: an updated systematic review. Ann Intern Med 2011;155(2):97–107.
28. Nutbeam D. The evolving concept of health literacy. Soc Sci Med 2008;67(12):2072–8.
29. Moore B, Stocks C, Owens P. Trends in emergency department visits, 2006–2014. Rockville (MD): Agency for Healthcare Research and Quality; 2017.
30. Fieldston E, Alpern E, Nadel F, et al. A qualitative assessment of reasons for nonurgent visits to the emergency department parent and health professional opinions. Pediatr Emerg Care 2012;28(3):220–5.
31. Morrison AK, Schapira MM, Gorelick MH, et al. Low caregiver health literacy is associated with higher pediatric emergency department use and nonurgent visits. Acad Pediatr 2014;14(3):309–14.
32. Yin HS, Johnson M, Mendelsohn AL, et al. The health literacy of parents in the United States: a nationally representative study. Pediatrics 2009;124(Supplement 3):S289–98.
33. Baker D, Stevens C, Brook R. Determinants of emergency department use by ambulatory patients at an urban public hospital. Ann Emerg Med 1995;25(3):311–6.
34. Yoffe SJ, Moore RW, Gibson JO, et al. A reduction in emergency department use by children from a parent educational intervention. Fam Med 2011;43(2):106.
35. Morrison AK, Myrvik MP, Brousseau DC, et al. The relationship between parent health literacy and pediatric emergency department utilization: a systematic review. Acad Pediatr 2013;13(5):421–9.
36. Senkomago V, Joseph R, Sierra M, et al. CDC activities to enhance training in cancer prevention and control in field epidemiology training programs in low- and middle-income countries. J Glob Oncol 2018;4:1–9.

Developing a Community Response

Collaborating Locally on Immigrant Care

Mary Brennan Wirshup, MD[a], Sarah Poutasse, RN, FNP-BC[a],
Adriana Deverlis, MPIA[b],*

KEYWORDS

- Immigrant health • Volunteer • Community partnership • Hispanic
- Fear of deportation • Hogar medico

KEY POINTS

- Many immigrant children have complex medical, dental, and behavioral health needs.
- Immigrant children typically do not choose to come to the United States, and they deserve to be healthy, happy, and pain-free regardless of their immigration status.
- Sustainable community responses to fostering immigrant health rely on creating a safe space for patients, a spirit of volunteerism, and strong community partnerships.
- In addition to medical, dental, and behavioral health care, culturally sensitive education is also an important part of providing effective care to immigrant patients.

INTRODUCTION

Give me your tired, your poor, your huddled masses yearning to breathe free, the wretched refuse of your teeming shore. Send these, the homeless, tempest-tost to me. I lift my lamp beside the golden door!
—(Lazarus, 1883, etched at the foot of the Statue of Liberty).

My passion for caring for immigrants started at the family dinner table when my father reminded us, 'never forget the poor and hungry, because we were poor and hungry.' My great-grandparents came to America from Ireland to escape starvation from the potato famine. My grandpa was the ice man, the door man, and the garbage man, and so when I look into the eyes of my patients, I see my family!
—(Dr. Mary Brennan Wirshup, author of this article).

Historically, the United States of America has welcomed immigrants from around the world. According to the Department of Homeland Security, more than 1 million

[a] Community Volunteers in Medicine, 300 Lawrence Drive, West Chester, PA 19380, USA; [b] Global Health Center, Children's Hospital of Philadelphia, 2716 South Street, 7th Floor, Station 7314, Philadelphia, PA 19146, USA
* Corresponding author.
E-mail address: deverlisa@email.chop.edu

Pediatr Clin N Am 66 (2019) 575–587
https://doi.org/10.1016/j.pcl.2019.02.006
0031-3955/19/© 2019 Elsevier Inc. All rights reserved.

people immigrated to the United States and obtained legal resident status in fiscal year 2017.[1] A recent review showed that an additional approximately 12 million undocumented immigrants resided in the United States in January 2014, with Mexico as the leading country of origin.[2]

Well into the 1900s, organized health care as we know it was virtually nonexistent in the United States, and medical care was limited to those who could readily afford it.[3] Churches and charitable groups often took up the mantle of caring for the poor and sick populations. The Samaritan Hospital, which was established by a minister in North Philadelphia in 1892 and later became Temple University Hospital, was an early example of charity care at its best. Samaritan Hospital provided free care to those in the poor and immigrant communities who were unable to pay, regardless of race, nationality, or creed.[4]

Despite health care advancements and new legislation, many low-income citizens continue to lack access to health care, especially the burgeoning immigrant population. The responsibility for taking care of this underserved population continues to fall on charity organizations, and Free Clinics have emerged to facilitate this care. The National Association of Free and Charitable Clinics reports that there are more than 1400 Free Clinics in the United States providing free medical care for those who are uninsured, underinsured, or have limited access to health care.[5] Some of these clinics are open just 1 day a week, offer limited services, or may operate from the basement of a church. Others, such as Community Volunteers in Medicine (CVIM) in West Chester, PA, are much more comprehensive, and may be associated with nearby medical schools or other nonprofit organizations. They are financed 100% by philanthropy.

Free Clinics use a volunteer/staff model to provide a range of medical, dental, pharmacy, vision, and behavioral health services. In return for meeting strict federal guidelines, they can provide free liability insurance to their largely volunteer, often retired, team of providers. In the early 1990s, the Volunteers in Medicine (VIM) organization created a model for the launch and operation of Free Clinics in a "Culture of Caring" environment that respects the dignity of the patient.

The 1400 Federally Qualified Health Centers (FQHCs) in the United States are another safety net that provides care to those who have limited resources or scarce health care alternatives. FQHC fees are charged on a sliding scale, they receive government support, and their patient eligibility criteria are less restrictive than for Free Clinics.[6,7] Public Health Departments are also answering the need of many immigrants by providing vaccinations, and screening and treatment for tuberculosis. This is so important for the community at large because it improves herd immunity and prevents dissemination of treatable disease.

This article describes CVIM's role in caring for the immigrant population of one region, as one of the 88 Free Clinics nationally using the VIM model.

At CVIM, we support the equal care of all adults and children in the United States, regardless of immigrant status.

CVIM is located 25 miles west of Philadelphia in Chester County, the wealthiest county in Pennsylvania (**Fig. 1**). According to the US Census Bureau's American Community Survey (2017), 47,128 immigrants reside in Chester County; nearly 5000 children younger than 18 years, and many of these children are our patients. Sixty-one percent of Chester County immigrants are Hispanic, mostly from Mexico, but also Ecuador, Guatemala, Venezuela, Honduras, and many other countries.[8]

The Committee on Community Health Services of the American Academy of Pediatrics defines immigrant children as "…those who are legal and illegal (undocumented) immigrants, refugees, and international adoptees."[9] We operate on the VIM principle that our "Culture of Caring" is inclusive and welcoming to all patients; each patient is

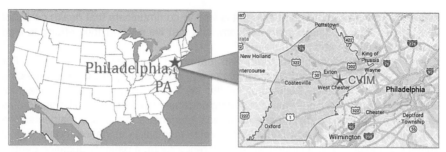

Fig. 1. Location of CVIM in Chester county near Philadelphia, Pennsylvania in the United States.

treated with respect and dignity.[10] The VIM model is extremely welcoming to immigrants from all backgrounds.

As a Free Clinic, we receive no federal funding or insurance, and we provide free care and medicine to working poor patients who do not have health insurance. Approximately two-thirds of CVIM patients speak Spanish as their primary language (**Fig. 2**). Although few of our providers are bilingual, we have a revolving team of nearly 40 volunteer interpreters and approximately one-half of our staff is fluent in Spanish, so language assistance is always available for appointments on-site.

This article describes the elements that make the community response by CVIM and other organizations most effective. The article draws on examples from CVIM's medical, dental, and behavioral health care services, and provides case studies to illustrate the unique challenges often faced by pediatric immigrant patients and how we work around those challenges. We hope that this model may be a helpful resource to other pediatric providers who serve similar populations across the United States and in other settings around the world.

DISCUSSION
Elements of Sustainability

There are 3 key factors to ensure the sustainability of an effective community response to caring for immigrant children: a safe space, funding and staff, and local partnerships. The first and primary factor in successfully providing quality care to immigrant children is to create a safe space that meets the holistic health needs of our patients. At a time in which the fear of deportation is real and constant, immigrant patients need to know that their clinics are safe places to receive excellent care. Messages of privacy and confidentiality are conveyed by word of mouth within immigrant communities, and reinforced in-person at the time of a patient's first encounter with CVIM

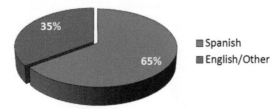

Fig. 2. Primary language spoken by CVIM patients.

staff, often during eligibility screening. It is vital to communicate that *health care, not immigration status, is our primary concern*, and that we support their efforts to lead productive, healthy, and hopeful lives.[11]

The way that a clinic is structured also matters in communicating this point. For example, CVIM is an integrated medical home, *Hogar Médico* in Spanish, providing comprehensive medical, behavioral health, and dental care all under one roof (**Fig. 3**). This creates opportunities for interdisciplinary learning and collaboration, as well as a fertile training experience for clinical students and medical residents. See **Fig. 4** for an example of how CVIM incorporates medical examination rooms, dental chairs and radiographs, a laboratory, a conference room, a patient education center, and education and counseling rooms into one facility.[12,13]

Second, it is important to have funding and staffing from a body of committed people and partners. A strong spirit of giving is key to the success and sustainability of this type of community response. When funding is tight, as it often is with philanthropic organizations like CVIM, it is crucial to make creative use of a small but strong core staff, combined with a wide range of clinical and support volunteers. The volunteer staff can be quite extensive; for example, CVIM has a team of more than 400 clinical and support volunteers, including more than 30 provider specialties, helping to ensure that the organization can provide comprehensive quality care.[14]

Third, yet perhaps most importantly for sustainability, effective community response requires beneficial and enduring partnerships with other local health care organizations and facilities, as well as with schools and faith communities, such as churches, to identify patients in need of services and to coordinate their care, no matter how complex their problems may be. Community partnerships enable organizations to provide the best possible care to patients by fostering a neighbors-helping-neighbors environment. Partnerships with other nonprofit hospitals and clinics can be leveraged to seek additional studies and expertise beyond what we can provide in-house. For CVIM, these institutions ensure that our patients get blood work, radiographs, computed tomography scans, MRIs, specialty consults, and even surgeries, all at no cost to the patients.

The Importance of Language Access

Even with these 3 elements in place, we cannot be truly accessible to immigrant patients if we cannot communicate effectively with them. Indeed, one of the biggest

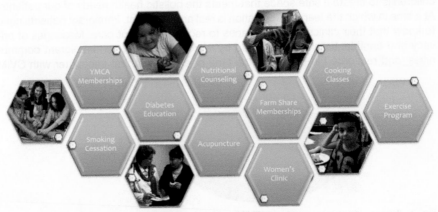

Fig. 3. A variety of programs are offered at CVIM.

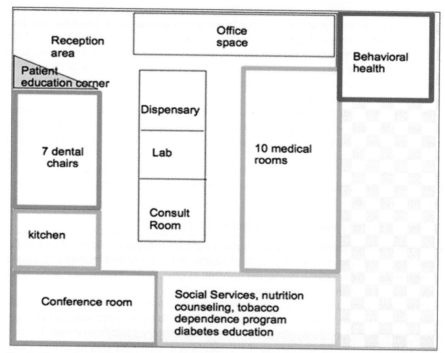

Fig. 4. Floor plan of CVIM's medical home.

obstacles in caring for immigrant medical, dental, and behavioral health patients is that many of them have limited English proficiency (LEP), creating unique challenges to patient-provider communication. Traditionally, LEP patients have relied on the providing organization's staff members with some degree of familiarity with a patient's preferred language, third-party telephone interpreter services, or patient family members.[15] It is particularly disconcerting when children of LEP caregivers are relied on to act as interpreters for their parents, even in their own clinical assessment.

Untrained medical interpretation has been associated with a higher likelihood of errors due to miscommunication. These errors include, but are not limited to, addition and omission errors in which interpreters modify provider or patient comments either by including additional phrases or leaving out words altogether.[16] Similarly, clinicians who are not trained to work well with interpreters can also cause problems in patient communication.

This can be avoided by maintaining a seasoned team of trained volunteer interpreters who are available to accompany LEP patient families throughout their visits. By having professional interpreters who are familiar with medical terminology and skilled at appropriate communication techniques, such as asking providers to repeat or rephrase statements made during an examination if they feel that patients have not understood the information that was intended to be conveyed, one can not only provide better care for LEP patients, but also help the patients and families to feel more confident in the care they receive.

Furthermore, all medical staff should be trained in how to work most effectively with interpreters. At CVIM, for example, we train clinicians to speak directly to the patient and not to the interpreter, which can undermine the desired provider–patient relationship. They are instructed to speak in short phrases to allow time for interpretation, and they are made aware that anything spoken in the examination room will be translated to the patient, so they must be cautious in what they say out loud. Likewise, our providers are reminded that their patients may possess a higher comprehension of the English language than they realize, so they should not speak under the assumption that the patient will not be able to understand. All of these are best practices to foster the most correct and professional communication between the patient (or their parents) and the provider (**Fig. 5**).

Interpreters allow the focus to be on the care of the pediatric patients, without burdening the child with the responsibility of interpreting their own examination or risking errors caused by their parents' limited English. Proper interpretation ensures that information about the medical problem and the education given to the patient's family about follow-up care is completely understood. As a result, at CVIM, families with LEP confidently interact with providers through the interpreters, ensuring the best possible outcomes (**Fig. 6**).

Challenges in Accessing Appropriate Medical Care

Ensuring that immigrant patients can access the care that they need requires a multifaceted approach to clinical care. Lack of insurance coverage and inadequate access to regular health care place immigrant children at greater risk for physical and mental health issues than their nonimmigrant counterparts.

Immigrant communities often lack basic health education; it is crucial that the health risks to these communities be explored and understood by both providers and the patients' parents or guardians, who often have an elementary education or less. The current political climate, which makes visits fraught with worry, as well as other cultural factors, contribute to less frequent medical care for immigrant children.[17]

In addition to routine childhood illnesses, some of the most common medical health problems in immigrant pediatric patients seen at CVIM include obesity, incomplete immunizations, exposure to tuberculosis, and asthma. Because many patients come from areas of the world in which tuberculosis remains prevalent, health care providers should establish a protocol for identifying those potentially affected and refer them to the local Health Department for tuberculosis exposure testing and for treatment if positive. The Health Department also provides free vaccinations to needy families (and testing for human immunodeficiency virus for uninsured adults); this important partnership means that we do not need to spend our limited resources on a service that is already available in the community.

Obesity is a significant public health concern in the United States, and it poses a particular challenge to immigrant and nonwhite children. From 2015 to 2016 in the United States, the overall prevalence of pediatric obesity was 18.5%, but the rates among black and Hispanic children (22% and 25.8%, respectively) underscore the

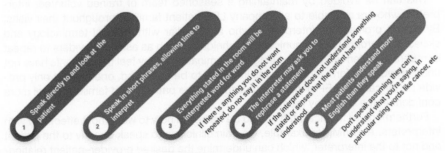

Fig. 5. CVIM's top 5 tips for working with interpreters.

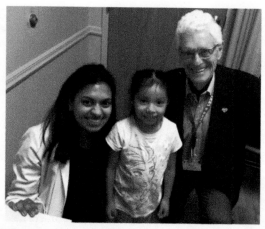

Fig. 6. One of CVIM's interpreters assisting during a patient visit.

importance of focusing on wellness in our patient community.[18] Obesity in our patient population is often driven by lack of knowledge, limited finances, and difficulty accessing healthy food, so clinical care must be coupled with education. To encourage healthy eating and increased nutritional knowledge among patients, we highly recommend including dieticians and nutrition counselors as part of the staff. At CVIM, we offer one-on-one counseling in nutrition and diabetes self-management, as well as cooking classes to help patients adopt healthier lifestyles (**Figs. 7** and **8**).

The importance of regular well-visit health examinations for children is also not well understood in most immigrant and refugee populations. Immigrant families are typically accustomed to episodic, infrequent health care that sends them to emergency rooms.[9] Effective community medical care for these patients must include education that encourages healthy behavior. For example, at the first pediatric visit at CVIM, we teach parents that they now have a *Hogar Médico* ("medical home"). We stress the importance of well-visits for their children to prevent illness as much as possible, and allow for early detection and treatment before an illness becomes emergent.

Medical Case Studies at Community Volunteers in Medicine

Many of CVIM's patients present with significant medical challenges that require multiple levels of care coordination. One such case was a 6-year-old boy from Venezuela, who immigrated 4 months before his first visit. His mother brought in his medical

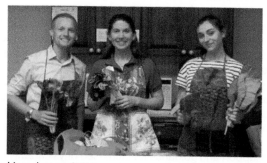

Fig. 7. Healthy cooking class at CVIM.

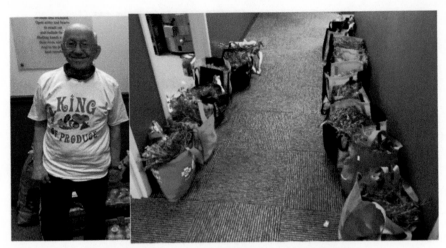

Fig. 8. Produce-sharing at CVIM for supplementing nutritional education.

records, which showed a history of precocious puberty; he had been taking a medication called leuprolide but had not had access to it for 4 months. As with any new patient at CVIM, our volunteer pediatrician documented a detailed history and performed a thorough physical examination. Because he required unique and specialized care beyond the scope of a family practice office, we were able to refer him to a nearby children's hospital, where they have a wonderful charity care program. They made it possible for this child to get the care he needed, and they will be able to provide care until he is 18. He was also referred to the Health Department for free immunizations, another one of our great partnerships. Thanks to these strong partnerships, we are able to help connect him and all of our patients with the treatment that they need.

Another recent case involved a 5-year-old child who had immigrated to the United States from Mexico at 2 years old. Her family of 4 was subletting a single room in a small apartment. For the past month, her mother had noted a very pruritic rash starting on her hands, which had spread to the rest of her body; the mom had also noted a similar rash on herself and her other children. On physical examination, she was found to have an extensive erythematous, maculopapular rash on her extremities and trunk, with obvious burrows and excoriations on the hands. The whole family was diagnosed with scabies, which is common in resource-poor communities,[19] and were all prescribed permethrin, a medication that our dispensary does not routinely stock. The least expensive prescription we could find using a discount prescription card service would still cost approximately $40 per patient, which they could not afford. CVIM purchased a small amount of an alternate treatment, ivermectin, and then successfully requested the manufacturer to donate the remaining medication. The family was given this prescription for free, and they completed the course of medication.

A third case arose from a routine physical of a 17-year-old Hispanic boy, whose main complaint was of a brown discoloration on his neck that he "could not wash off." On examination, he was found to have a body mass index of 32.5 and was diagnosed with typical acanthosis nigricans. He had a strong family history of diabetes, with his father being insulin-dependent, so we referred him for laboratory work to determine if he might have diabetes or prediabetes. We also referred him to our nutritionist for dietary support and guidance for increased physical activity. As we cared for him, we involved his mother, who does the family's shopping and cooking, in his care.

Dental Care Among Immigrant Populations

It is important to recognize the unique dental needs among immigrant children and work with the community to respond. For instance, dental issues are particularly prevalent among Mexican-American immigrant children. According to *Healthy People 2010*,[20] 43% of Hispanic children aged 6 to 8 have untreated caries, compared with 36% of non-Hispanic black children and 26% of non-Hispanic white children. Many immigrant children present with extensive cavities and often painful mouth abscesses, and it takes many visits to treat these acute issues before preventive care can be addressed. Children may miss many hours of school because of dental issues. In addition, children cannot learn when in pain, so it is crucial that these issues are taken seriously.

In addition to seeing children who come into the clinic, it is important to proactively identify patients who are in need of care but have not yet been reached. This can be done by collaborating with local school nurses and school dental hygienists to identify children with dental issues and then getting parental permission to bring the students from school to the clinic. One might also consider working with schools to initiate programs to provide fluoride varnish to children.

Culturally sensitive parent education is another important part of the dental care puzzle. A common problem among immigrant children is early childhood caries due to excessive bottle use, as many parents continue to put older infants and young toddlers to sleep with a bottle of milk or juice. A study of urban Mexican-American mothers showed that only approximately one-half knew that this use of infant bottles was a primary cause of their child's caries.[21] In addition to teaching on this subject, it is also recommended to teach parents about the importance of starting dental care for their children at age 1, and about the importance of preventive dental care. As health care providers, we must recognize the knowledge deficits in the immigrant population and provide culturally sensitive education to improve each child's oral health (**Figs. 9** and **10**).

Dental Case Studies at Community Volunteers in Medicine

A recent pediatric dental case demonstrates the severity of dental issues seen at CVIM. A 5-year-old Portuguese immigrant was referred to us from Head Start because of mouth pain. At CVIM, our pediatric dentist's initial assessment revealed 9 cavities and an abscess. Silver Diamine Fluoride (SDF) drops were put on the cavities to prevent progression until care could be arranged. The cost of one 200-drop SDF bottle is $125; 1 drop treats up to 5 teeth. We use these drops frequently because they are an extremely cost-effective method of arresting tooth decay for patients like him. He was also started on antibiotics, and then, due to the extent of his dental issues, he was referred to the outpatient dental surgery center for $6000 worth of procedures under

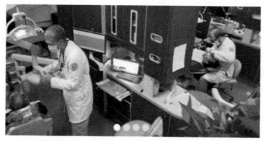

Fig. 9. Two of our 7 dental operatories in use.

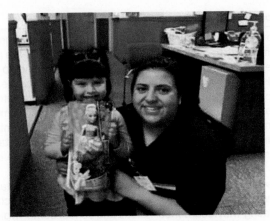

Fig. 10. One of our pediatric dental patients receiving extra care.

anesthesia. The head of our dental program researched and secured a foundation grant to care for him. Now that this is all done, he will start on preventive care and is on the path to great dental health in the future.

Another recent case involved a 7-year-old Mexican immigrant, who presented with significant discomfort and was found to have a dental abscess among other dental problems. At her first visit, antibiotics were started and an extraction was scheduled for the next visit. Over the next several months, she also had 7 cavities filled and 4 sealants applied, all at CVIM. Her follow-up visit revealed that she is now cavity-free, pain-free, and able to learn and play like any other child.

Unique Behavioral Health Care Needs

Finally, there are many important behavioral health issues and psychological stressors that are unique to immigrant patients. Many patients are afraid to leave their homes due to the current political climate, leading to cancellations of much-needed appointments.

Frequently, the issue of trauma also needs to be addressed. Many patients have suffered physically and psychologically in their country of origin or as they traveled to the United States. Some have fled persecution or danger in their home country. Others came to the United States and found themselves involved in intimate partner violence situations. The immigrant population is more likely to stay in these abusive relationships because of the vulnerability caused by their immigration status, as well as cultural norms that discourage them from reporting abuse. The exposure of their children to this abuse contributes to an accumulation of adverse childhood experiences that, if not addressed, can impact their health and behavior for a lifetime.[22]

Issues of violence and abuse scar patients emotionally and can interfere with their well-being. However, immigrant populations are often less likely to seek mental health care because of their cultural backgrounds, which stigmatize mental health issues. To assist our patients, CVIM has both a social services coordinator and a behavioral health coordinator on-site, both bilingual. We were also able to secure a grant to expand our behavioral health services because the needs of our population are so great and community resources are so limited.

Immigrant issues and cultural differences in parenting styles also present challenges to patients as parents. They work long hours under heavy stress, and they are not able to use the physical approaches to discipline they have relied on once they come to the

United States. Parenting support classes designed to provide parenting style alternatives and coping skills for immigrant parents are a helpful approach to combat this challenge.

Behavioral Health Case Studies at Community Volunteers in Medicine

One recent behavioral health case that reflects the adolescent immigrant experience of our patients is a teenage girl, who immigrated to Chester County with her parents when she was 3 years old. Her mother abandoned the family the following year; her father works 7 days a week and struggles with alcoholism. She was raised in her uncle's house, where she was neglected and abused. Two years ago, she was diagnosed with bipolar 1 disorder with psychotic features, complicated by drug and alcohol addictions. Her father was recently deported, so this patient, now in high school, lives at a friend's house. She is currently going through a coordinated care regimen at CVIM in which she sees our staff counselor weekly and one of our volunteer psychiatrists every 3 months. We provide her free medication through our dispensary. Without this coordinated care, she would likely be headed toward the juvenile justice system and psychiatric admissions without hope of breaking this cycle.

She now has new anxiety issues as she is making plans for after high school. She dreams of attending college, but her legal status remains uncertain. Many of our young patients continue to dream of a better life despite their barriers, and we are dedicated to providing them many levels of coordinated care to help facilitate their dreams.

Another story at our clinic is that of a young couple, who have faced many challenges as child immigrants. The young man was born in Central America to a very large family. His father was physically abusive and neglectful, and his mother struggled to provide for her children, forcing the older children to work at very young ages for minimal pay. He explained that in his country, there was little opportunity to make money except through drug trafficking, and he was determined to escape the violence of his home and his country. As a teenager, he made the journey north into the United States to find ways to help his mother with financial support and to seek better opportunities for himself. On arrival, he worked hard to complete high school with good grades and eventually received asylum in the United States, where he has aspirations to continue his studies. He is now an adult and works long hours to support himself, his girlfriend, and his family back home.

His girlfriend, also a CVIM patient, was born in another Latin American country to a mentally ill mother who was inconsistently present in her life, and who eventually moved to the United States without her children. Our patient spent much of her childhood caring for her 2 younger half-sisters. She and her sisters traveled to the United States to be with their mother, who then left her the full responsibilities of the house, while continuing to bounce from one relationship to the next. Our patient became more depressed after moving to the United States, feeling isolated from her extended family and her culture, and struggling to catch up academically. One day, to her shock, her mother sold her to 2 men who raped her. She began using drugs and alcohol to cope with the pain and betrayal.

This young couple met as teenagers and they quickly fell in love. He encouraged her to stop using drugs and alcohol, work hard in school, and get out of her mother's house. With the assistance of protective services and legal support, she emancipated herself from her mother and moved into an apartment with her boyfriend. She was granted asylum in the United States her senior year of high school.

Both patients now see our counselor as they plan to get married and hope to gain custody of her 2 younger siblings. They are resilient, determined young adults who are working to address their childhood traumas, both recent and in the distant past. They have experienced great relief in sharing the intimate details of their past traumas in therapy, and continue to seek support and closure through counseling here at CVIM.

SUMMARY

Dr Fernando Stein, MD, FAAP, former president of the American Academy of Pediatrics, issued his "Statement on Protecting Immigrant Children" in 2017, noting that "The mission of the American Academy of Pediatrics is to protect the health and well-being of all children, no matter where they or their parents were born."[23] Many communities have immigrant children with limited resources and complex medical, dental, and behavioral health needs. These children did not choose to come here, and they deserve to be healthy, happy, and pain-free no matter their situation.

Developing an effective community response to the health care needs (medical, dental, and behavioral) of immigrant children and families requires several key elements. To be successful and sustainable, Free Clinics like CVIM must create a safe, accessible environment for patients, have a reliable and dedicated group of core staff, many volunteers, and dedicated donors, and develop a breadth of strong community partnerships. They must provide holistic care that takes into account the patients' contexts and histories, and this care must be accessible to them in their own language through independent, qualified interpreters and from medical staff trained to work effectively with these interpreters. Care must address not only medical needs but also dental and behavioral health, and take into account a multitude of unique challenges that immigrant patients may face.

"Until I came to CVIM, I did not realize how much my neighbors were suffering. My hope is that one of these children will go to medical school and take my place, taking care of the next generation of immigrants. In that way, the inscription etched into that great Statue of Liberty will continue to inspire hope for future generations of Americans." – Dr Wirshup.

ACKNOWLEDGMENTS

Alberta Landis, Miriam Geiger, Edgar Weyback-Liogier, Meghan McDonald, Jane Orner.

REFERENCES

1. U.S. Department of Homeland Security. Legal immigration and adjustment of status report fiscal year 2017, quarter 4. 2018. In: Yearbook of immigration statistics. 2017. Available at: https://www.dhs.gov/immigration-statistics/special-reports/legal-immigration. Accessed September 10, 2018.
2. Baker B. Estimates of the unauthorized immigrant population residing in the United States: January 2014. DHS Office of Immigration Statistics, Office of Strategy, Policy & Plans; 2017. p. 1–9. Available at: https://www.dhs.gov/sites/default/files/publications/Unauthorized%20Immigrant%20Population%20Estimates%20in%20the%20US%20January%202014_1.pdf.
3. Griffin J. The history of healthcare in America. In: JP Griffin Group, editor 2017. Available at: https://www.griffinbenefits.com/employeebenefitsblog/history_of_healthcare. Accessed December 3, 2018.
4. Mission & History. In: Temple University hospital system. Available at: https://tuh.templehealth.org/content/mission.htm. Accessed December 3, 2018.
5. NAFC Clinics. America's free and charitable clinics: vital support for 30 million uninsured Americans 2013. Available at: http://www.nafcclinics.org/sites/

default/files/NAFC%20Infographic%20%26%20Report%20Feb%202%202015%20small.pdf. Accessed December 3, 2018.

6. FCQH germane: effective FQHC & medicaid strategies. What is an FQHC?. Available at: https://www.fqhc.org/what-is-an-fqhc/. Accessed December 3, 2018.

7. Department of Health and Human Services. [Infographic] Federally Qualified Health Center. Available at: https://static1.squarespace.com/static/53023 f77e4b0f0275ec6224a/t/5a29875a0d92972420c91437/1512671067129/fqhcfa ctsheet.pdf. Accessed December 3, 2018.

8. U.S. Census Bureau. 2012-2016 American community survey 5-year estimates: selected characteristics of the native and foreign-born populations, Chester County, Pennsylvania. 2017. Available at: https://factfinder.census.gov/faces/tableservices/jsf/pages/productview.xhtml?src=CF. Accessed October 10, 2018.

9. Committee on Community Health Services. Health care for children of immigrant families. Pediatrics 1997;100(1):153–6.

10. Volunteers in Medicine. VIM model. Available at: http://vimdev.zendata.me/vim-model/. Accessed September 10, 2018.

11. Volunteers in Medicine. History and mission. Available at: http://volunteersinmedicine.org/about-us/history-and-mission-health-care-clinics/. Accessed September 10, 2018.

12. Community Volunteers in Medicine. Mission & vision. Available at: http://cvim.org/about-us/staff/. Accessed September 10, 2018.

13. Community Volunteers in Medicine. [Infographic] Fiscal year 2017 highlights. 2017. Available at: http://cvim.org/wp-content/uploads/2016/03/FY17-Highlights_Infographics-Full-Page-1.pdf. Accessed September 10, 2018.

14. Community Volunteers in Medicine. Staff. Available at: http://cvim.org/about-us/staff/. Accessed September 10, 2018.

15. Partridge R, Proano L. Communicating with immigrants: medical interpreters in health care. Med Health 2010;93(3):77–8.

16. Flores G, Laws B, Mayo SJ, et al. Errors in medical interpretation and their potential clinical consequences in pediatric encounters. Pediatrics 2003;111(1):6–14.

17. Huang ZJ, Yu SM, Ledsky R. Health status and health service access and use among children in U.S. immigrant families. Am J Public Health 2006;96(4): 634–40.

18. Hales CM, Carroll MD, Fryar CD, et al. Prevalence of obesity among adults and youth: United States, 2015-2016. NCHS data brief, no 288. Hyattsville (MD): National Center for Health Statistics; 2017.

19. World Health Organization. Lymphatic filariasis. 2018. Available at: http://www.who.int/lymphatic_filariasis/epidemiology/scabies/en. Accessed June 14, 2018.

20. Centers for Disease Control and Prevention. Healthy people 2010. Available at: https://www.cdc.gov/nchs/healthy_people/hp2010.htm. Accessed December 10, 2018.

21. Hoeft KS, Barker JC, Masterson EE. Urban Mexican-American mothers' beliefs about caries etiology in children. 2010. Available at: https://www.ncbi.nlm.nih.gov/pmc/articles/PMC3600053/. Accessed June 14, 2018.

22. Centers for Disease Control and Prevention. Adverse childhood experiences (ACEs). 2016. Available at: https://www.cdc.gov/violenceprevention/acestudy/index.html. Accessed November 12, 2018.

23. Stein Fernando, MD, FAAP, President, American Academy of Pediatrics AAP statement on protecting immigrant children 1/25/2017. Available at: https://www.aap.org/en-us/about-the-aap/aap-press-room/Pages/AAPStatementonProtectingImmigrant Children.aspx. Accessed November 12, 2018.

Clinical Tools for Working Abroad with Migrants

Ryan McAuley, MD, MPH

KEYWORDS

- Refugee health care • Migrant health care • Disaster response
- Humanitarian assistance

KEY POINTS

- The provision of health care services to migrants abroad is challenging and dynamic and requires a public health approach.
- Many factors contribute to the health status of migrants along their journey.
- Clinical and public health priorities for migrants require coordination and collaboration between partner agencies and host countries.
- There is a listing of migrant health online resources for various international agencies, international nongovernmental organizations, and universities.
- A practical guide for health care professionals seeking experience with migrant health care in the field is provided.

INTRODUCTION

At the end of 2017, there were an estimated 68.5 million forcibly displaced people worldwide, of whom about one-half are children under the age of 18 years.[1] Of these, an estimated 20,000 unaccompanied minors or separated children arrived in European countries as migrants in 2017.[2] These numbers are staggering and the individual health needs of this cohort are dynamic and challenging. Many complex factors contribute to the health status of individual migrants, but often an individualized approach to clinical care is not feasible owing to resource limitations, a lack of trained personnel, and access barriers.

Providing health care for migrants abroad requires a public health approach that makes the most of limited resources and strives to incorporate nuances of a relevant social and cultural framework. There are many variables that affect the strategy of such an intervention. Consider the following 3 examples of unique migrant groups:

- *Rohingya migrants in Bangladesh*[3]: A large and rapidly expanding group of migrants from a common ethnic minority group in Rakhine State, Myanmar.

Disclosure Statement: No disclosures.
Division of Hematology/Oncology, Department of Medicine, University of Pennsylvania Perelman School of Medicine, 10th Floor, South Pavilion, Room 10-165, 3400 Civic Center Boulevard, Philadelphia, PA 19104, USA
E-mail address: ryan.mcauley@uphs.upenn.edu

Hundreds of thousands of migrants fled their homes in a massive exodus after violent clashes began in August 2017. They settled in a densely populated camp in the southern part of Bangladesh where the infrastructure was never meant to accommodate such a large number of people in such a short period of time.

- *Bhutanese refugees in Nepal*[4]*:* An ethnic minority group fled to Nepal decades ago and was dispersed in several chronic, stable camp settings without much movement in or out. Multiple generations of children have been born to migrant parents and have grown up in displacement. A resettlement campaign was launched in 2007 with a coalition of countries accepting these migrants as refugees. Since then, more than 100,000 migrants have been resettled out of Nepal to other countries of asylum around the world.
- *Internally displaced persons (IDPs) in South Sudan*[5,6]*:* As of September 2018, there are an estimated 1.84 million people displaced within South Sudan. The newest country on the planet has been plagued by a civil war that began in December 2013. The number of displaced persons throughout the country has varied depending on conflict hotspots, relative vulnerability of ethnic groups, and food insecurity. The displaced groups are not uniform and there are differences in ethnicity, areas of origin, the areas that are sought for refuge, and the duration of time spent internally displaced versus crossing a border to a neighboring country.

HEALTH AND DISPLACEMENT

The health status of migrants is unique and complex with many dynamic variables. First, simply being displaced from one's home can lead to a wide array of potential health consequences. The duration of time and experiences leading up to displacement also has an effect on health. The effects of well-established biopsychosocial determinants of health must also be considered. The potential downstream health effects of all these variables combined are wide-ranging in potential scope and severity.

When contrasting different migrant experiences, there is a continuum of time with regard to the lead-up to actual displacement, the distance required for transit, and the time it takes to reach one's destination. This timeline can be influenced by a myriad of factors ranging from fear of attack to socioeconomic status to geopolitical factors. At the core, there is a range of personal resilience factors that lead to an individual or family's decision that "enough is enough" and that leaving one's home is a better option than staying in it.

First, consider a village under sudden aerial missile attack by a powerful opponent. In this type of acute and violent situation, loud and destructive ordinances lead to immediate feelings of vulnerability, loss of control, and fear, which can be far-reaching from the actual points of impact. Some people in the village will be killed directly as a result of the explosions. Others will decide to shelter in place, perhaps in their own home or with friends and family who may be in safer areas of the village. Still others will decide to swiftly and immediately flee the village altogether. In this acute situation, migrants do not have time to collect valuables, or significant food or clothing, or other livelihood items. They may not be able to go far (ie, crossing a border), but they must flee swiftly to escape the immediate threat of danger. They grab their children and go.

Second, consider a more protracted situation in a country where the national government is failing and the political situation devolves over several years. During this time, opposition forces may gain strength in different parts of the country against a weakened government military. As areas of the country are conquered by rebel insurgents, the people living in those areas may be forced to comply with extremist religious or cultural practices, or else face harsh violence, torture, or even death. Some people in this situation will fully comply with the new laws and social norms and may even be recruited to join the insurgent forces. At the opposite extreme, other people may completely resist the new ruling structure and stand their ground even in the face of dire consequences. These people may be killed and become martyrs for their beliefs. Or they may experience severe violence and then become compliant. Or, they may experience severe violence and decide to flee. In the middle between these extremes, there will potentially be a much larger group of people who temporarily adapt to the new rules to protect life and loved ones and intend to maintain a low profile. They will try to continue life as they know it, compromising some values and freedoms to stay in their homes and near their family, friends, and community. Perhaps they will set limits of restrictions they will not comply with, that is, "if the rebels force child marriage, then we will take our young girls and flee." Or they will set time-sensitive limits, that is, "we will save our money in case government forces do not regain control in the next 12 months so that we can flee." Or perhaps they will reach a breaking point unexpectedly that triggers the desire to flee. In all of these scenarios, the time to displacement is longer than the first example. These migrants need more time to plan and research their route and save money and resources. They are forced to weigh the risks of staying with the risks of fleeing and compromised safety along the way. There may not be an immediate threat to life and livelihood, but there might be a persistently growing discord that can involve psychological and/or physical trauma. They must balance a difficult equation: how much of X can I endure to maintain Y?

For migrant children, there are many potential effects of displacement on normal childhood behavior and development.[7,8] Aside from the direct effects of stress and trauma on children and their parents, there are a multitude of other dynamics that may be difficult to quantify or evaluate. Consider a family in the first scenario, sheltering in place in village that is under attack for months at a time. Small children may not have opportunities to play outside, run, explore, or play with other children. School-age children may not be able to attend school because it is not safe to do so, the teachers have fled or, the school is closed or damaged. In the second scenario, teenagers may have to halt their education prematurely to work and contribute to the family's income. While in transit, families may not be able to enroll their children in local schools out of fear of deportation or restricted access. Immigration authorities may detain transiting migrant families in detention centers or prisons for weeks, months, or years. At the time of writing, there is a lack of peer-reviewed research investigating the potential effects of detention on child development and behavior. However, one can surmise that physical confinement and institutional stress cannot have a positive effect on how children learn and grow. Unaccompanied minors in transit are particularly vulnerable to exploitation, trafficking, and interrupted education.[2,9] Last, children may experience further difficulty by shifting languages in their home country, in transit, and in the country of destination, which will further impair their learning and social development.[8]

There are biopsychosocial determinants of health which are not unique to displacement, but compound the health stresses of displacement and affect resilience. Consider the following list of examples:

- Family size and age of children
- Economic status
- Education level: skilled versus unskilled labor
- Health status: chronic diseases; endemic diseases in source, transit, and destination countries; access to health care systems

- Mental health: trauma reactions, mood disorders, toxic stress, developmental delay
- Immunization status
- Sanitation and hygiene standards: source country versus transit versus destination
- Environmental stress: temperature extremes, limited clothing, inadequate shelter, access to clean water, exposure to tobacco smoke and biofuels
- Nutrition: access to adequate food in the source country versus transit versus the destination
- Duration of transit/migration
- Travel hazards[10]: road, boat, train accidents

APPROACH TO PROVIDING HEALTH CARE SERVICES TO MIGRANTS ABROAD

Migrants face many health challenges along their journey. When structuring health care services for migrants abroad, there is not a one-size-fits-all approach and programming must be adaptable, practical, relevant, sustainable, and ideally integrated into the host country's health care system.

First, the goal of health care delivery for migrants abroad has to be defined in scope and purpose. For most migrants along their journey, the dynamic health challenges already discussed will not become stabilized or improved until a migrant has reached a permanent or semipermanent destination. This also assumes that migrants will have access to existing health care systems in the destination country. However, this is often not the case. One example is IDPs in South Sudan. Owing to many years of ongoing conflict and instability, South Sudan has a completely overwhelmed and nonfunctional public health care system. For the 1.84 million IDPs in South Sudan who are seeking refuge from active fighting, most are unable to access functioning government health care structures.[11] Both IDPs and host populations in this context must rely heavily on nongovernmental organizations (NGOs) for health care and these organizations may not have a long-lasting presence or capacity to replace large-scale government services. Another common conundrum in health care provision for migrants is limited access to existing health care services in countries of transit or asylum. The pathway to refugee status and resettlement can take years, which is a long time for migrants struggling with unreliable healthcare access. In the early years of the Syrian civil war, displaced Syrians seeking refuge in neighboring countries throughout the Middle East and North Africa had difficulty accessing local health care services until more inclusive policies were put into place.[12]

To complicate matters for many migrants around the world, displacement often becomes the destination. There are many geopolitical factors that can lead to this stagnation along the migration route from home country to transit country to country of asylum to country of destination or resettlement. The effects can be seen in long-standing refugee camps (ie, Dadaab and Kakuma in Kenya) where multiple generations of families have lived for years and children are born and raised in camp settings.[13,14] These children grow up far away from the traditional homes of their parents and grandparents, under the auspices of protection from the United Nations (UN), and in settings that were never intended for long-term settlement or typical societies.

In all of these examples, there is a crucial role for a public health approach to the provision of health care services for migrants. Simply put, there should be a common objective to decrease morbidity and mortality, decrease suffering, and restore dignity for these vulnerable groups through a package of services incorporating curative and preventive care. We must also recognize the reality of resource limitations with regard to this goal. Host countries are often not inclined to invest in resources for migrant groups who might only be transiting through their country and not effectively contributing to the economy. Often, health care services for migrants are provided through support from NGOs and local organizations. Thus, there has to be an approach for doing the most good for the most number of people with the resources available.

The overlap in clinical care and public health care is both codependent and synergistic in this situation. An emphasis on a single discipline without the other is impractical. This sort of horizontal and comprehensive approach can be a daunting task to establish, especially in areas affected by active conflict or mass displacement. Services are often bundled and divided among partner organizations based on operational agreements and mandates agreed on between organizations and a particular country or UN agency.[15] Advocacy with other partner organizations helps to highlight unmet needs and fill the gaps in service provision. No single organization is capable of providing a full package of services, and coordination and communication are essential, especially in humanitarian emergencies.

Clinical care priorities for migrants[16]

- Stabilization and curative approach for acute health conditions (acute illness, trauma, surgical emergencies)
- Screen and treat children and pregnant/lactating women for moderate and severe acute malnutrition
- Isolation and treatment of communicable diseases with outbreak potential (ie, measles, cholera)
- Realistic maintenance of chronic medical conditions (noncommunicable diseases)
- Full package of maternal–child health care (prenatal care, delivery care, emergency obstetric care, postnatal care, family planning, safe abortions)
- Sexual and gender-based violence case management (postexposure prophylaxis, emergency contraception, mental health, protection)
- Human immunodeficiency virus/tuberculosis screening and treatment programs
- Mental health and psychological first aid

Public health priorities[16]

- Vaccination against preventable diseases (ie, measles, polio, diphtheria, cholera, meningococcal meningitis)
- Access to clean water, sanitation, and hygiene
- Access to a stable food supply and adequate nutrition
- Disease monitoring, surveillance, and reporting
- Shelter, livelihood, and protection
- Community health education
- Coordination with other agencies and partner organizations

Not all migrants will fit neatly into one of these categories of illness or public health needs. Patients who present with complex medical conditions in resource-limited settings can present unique challenges for providers who rely on basic diagnostic tools and have limited referral capacity for more sophisticated evaluation and treatment. In acute humanitarian emergencies, basic triage protocols lead teams to focus attention and energy on patients who are not moribund and those who can be stabilized with presumably reversible or curable conditions. In more stable contexts, referrals to specialists might be possible, however, providers must balance the dynamics of the severity of disease, the prognosis, the availability of treatment and expertise of local professionals, the effectiveness based on available evidence, and the potential unintended consequences of additional stress on the family. For some of these complex clinical dilemmas, health care providers are forced to accept limitations and must help to reframe goals with migrant families. In some cases, a focus on symptom management, palliation, and an open discussion of prognosis and disease trajectory is the most appropriate treatment plan.

CLINICAL TOOLS AND RESOURCES FOR REFUGEE AND MIGRANT HEALTH CARE

The majority of health care professionals working with migrant populations abroad will have access to relevant clinical resources and guidelines specific to a particular agency, organization, country and/or population. The following sites have a wide range of resources, tools and research publications available for download. Although this is not an exhaustive list, it provides a framework for exploring available online resources in this rapidly-changing landscape. The list has been grouped by international agencies, international NGOs, and university and education-based organizations (Tables 1–3).

Table 1
International agency standards and guidelines

Organization	Website	Scope	Highlights
World Health Organization (WHO)	http://www.who.int/publications/guidelines/en/	International Regional Maternal/child health Nutrition Disease specific Health systems Patient safety Public health	List of essential drugs Nutrition guidelines Health care of children in humanitarian emergencies Outbreak management
UN High Commissioner for Refugees (UNHCR)	https://www.unhcr.org/resources-and-publications.html	International Regional Country specific Research Nutrition Sexual and reproductive health Mental health	UNHCR's essential medicines and medical supplies HIV in humanitarian emergencies Infant and young child feeding practices
International Organization for Migration (IOM)	http://publications.iom.int/	International Regional Policy/legal Child protection Trafficking Health	Migration health services medical manual Caring for trafficked persons
UNICEF	https://www.unicef.org/publications/	International Regional Policy Child protection Unaccompanied minors Health Nutrition Vaccination	A child is a child: protecting children on the move from violence, abuse and exploitation

(continued on next page)

Table 1 (continued)			
Organization	**Website**	**Scope**	**Highlights**
Centers for Disease Control and Prevention (CDC)	https://www.cdc.gov/ immigrantrefugeehealth/ index.html	International Disease specific Health screening Population-specific health profiles	Malaria guidelines Vaccination guidelines Technical guidelines for overseas medical examination
The Sphere Project	https://www. spherestandards.org/ resources/	International Policy Public health Water and sanitation Nutrition Health Child protection SGBV	The Sphere Handbook

Abbreviation: SGBV, sexual and gender-based violence.

Table 2 International NGOs			
Organization	Website	Scope	Highlights
Medecins Sans Frontieres/ Doctors Without Borders	http://refbooks.msf.org/ https://www.msf.org/	Clinical guidelines Refugee health Public health Maternal/Child Health	Clinical guidelines Essential drugs Tuberculosis guidelines Obstetric and newborn care
Save The Children	https://www. savethechildren.org/us/ about-us/resource-library/ health-library	Clinical guidelines Advocacy Policy guidelines Education resources Nutrition Water/ sanitation	Emergency health and nutrition toolkit Infant and young child feeding in emergencies toolkit
International Rescue Committee	https://www.rescue.org/ reports-and-resources	Clinical guidelines SGBV guidelines Nutrition Maternal/child health	Clinical care for sexual assault survivors (CCSAS)
International Committee of the Red Cross	https://www.icrc.org/en/ resource-centre	Clinical/surgical guidelines Public health Prison health Protection Mental health International humanitarian law	Guidelines on mental health and psychosocial support War and public health Health emergencies in large populations (H.E.L.P.)

Abbreviation: SGBV, gender-based violence.

Table 3
University-based and other resources

Organization	Website	Scope	Highlights
Relief Web	https://reliefweb.int/	Broad-based web site resource for humanitarian assistance and disaster response	Context updates Job postings Training Resources
Humanitarian U	https://humanitarianu.com/	Training Certification	Online training Field simulations
Johns Hopkins Bloomberg School of Public Health Center for Humanitarian Health	http:// hopkinshumanitarianhealth. org/	Broad-based university resource Masters of public health area of concentration	Refugee Health Disaster response Mental health Public health Research Education and training Open courseware
Columbia University Mailman School of Public Health Program on Forced Migration and Health	https://www.mailman. columbia.edu/research/ program-forced-migration- and-health	Broad-based university resource Masters of public health area of concentration	Refugee Health Disaster response Mental health Water and sanitation Maternal/child health Research Education and training
Harvard Humanitarian Initiative (HHI)	https://hhi.harvard.edu/	Broad-based university resource Interdisciplinary center of excellence	Humanitarian Academy at Harvard (HAH) Masters of public health concentration in humanitarian studies, ethics and human rights E-learning Workshops Research Human rights International humanitarian law

HOW TO GET INVOLVED IN MIGRANT HEALTH CARE ABROAD: A PRACTICAL GUIDE

Health care professionals seeking hands-on, practical experiences with migrant health care in the field have many options ranging in duration, context, and acuity. The breadth of options and variables can be daunting, and some will find it challenging to know where to begin and what to expect on the ground. Owing to the dynamic health disparities and challenges discussed in this article, there is usually a steep learning curve in the field, even for experienced providers. It takes time to understand the health needs, the cultural and political context, the resource limitations, and how to optimize care delivery within the framework of a particular organization or agency.

Choosing an organization or agency to partner with is a good starting point. NGOs tend to have a variety of short and long-term assignments. International agencies such as the UN, World Health Organization, and Centers for Disease Control and Prevention will tend to have long-term placement options only, but may also have short-term consulting opportunities for experienced professionals. The lead time can be lengthy for all of these options and human resource needs in the field can be dynamic and variable. A great deal of flexibility is required with regard to timing and this can be challenging for practicing health care workers to negotiate with their employers. Some aspects and variables to consider are listed.

CONSIDERATIONS IN CHOOSING AN ORGANIZATION FOR MIGRANT HEALTH CARE FIELDWORK

- Type of organization
  - International agency (World Health Organization, UN, Centers for Disease Control and Prevention)
  - International NGO (*Medecins Sans Frontieres*, Save the Children, International Rescue Committee)
  - Faith-based organizations (Samaritan's Purse, Catholic Relief Services)
  - University-based partnerships
- Mission, vision, and values
  - How well an individual's beliefs, ideals, and skill -set align with a particular organization or agency
  - Reputation and notoriety of the organization
  - Recognized partnerships
  - Specific mandates or areas of intervention
  - Neutrality and impartiality versus targeted response
    - Specific ethnic or religious group
    - One group involved in a conflict
    - Specific disease response or vertical program
- Timeline of organizational needs and availability for field work
  - Organization-specific
  - Variable human resource needs in the field
    - Need for prior humanitarian work experience
    - Rate of turnover for field workers
    - Programmatic changes: expanding, stable, or consolidating
    - Area of specialty/expertise of the health care professional
    - Foreign language skills
    - Nationality/relevant travel restrictions
- Duration of intended fieldwork: short term (weeks to months) versus long term (months to years)
- Organization or agency funding source
  - Independent funding
  - Special interests including potential conflicts of interest (government funding, restricted funds or programs, pharmaceutical industry funding)
- Security context
  - Highly variable depending on specific location
  - Must clearly understand security management approach of specific organizations
  - Should have an awareness of
    - Security stakeholders in the field and in the headquarters
    - Chain of command and communication
    - Capacity and procedure for emergency evacuation

- o Informed approach to personal security risks versus organizational risks and how each are appropriately mitigated
- Professional liability: malpractice insurance coverage for specific profession
- Staff health in the field
  - o Understand the capacity and reputation of the organization for taking care of health needs of field-worker staff
    - ■ Predeparture health care
    - ■ Access to standard personal protective equipment in field
    - ■ Confidentiality of staff health care services in the field
    - ■ Capacity for emergency medical evacuation
    - ■ Psychosocial support for field workers before, during, and after missions
- Financial considerations
  - o Salaries, stipends, benefits (travel, housing, health care insurance, meals), pro bono volunteer work

REFERENCES

1. United Nations High Commissioner for Refugees. UNHCR global trends in forced displacement 2017. 2018.
2. UNICEF. Latest statistics and graphics on refugee and migrant children: latest information on children arriving in Europe. Available at: https://www.unicef.org/eca/emergencies/latest-statistics-and-graphics-refugee-and-migrant-children. Accessed December 18, 2018.
3. The United Nations High Commissioner for Refugees. UNHCR: Bangladesh Rohingya emergency. Available at: https://www.unhcr.org/ph/campaigns/rohingya-emergency. Accessed December 18, 2018.
4. Shrestha DD. Resettlement of Bhutanese refugees surpasses 100,000 mark 2015. Available at: https://www.unhcr.org/news/latest/2015/11/564dded46/resettlement-bhutanese-refugees-surpasses-100000-mark.html. Accessed December 18, 2018.
5. The United Nations High Commissioner for Refugees. UNHCR: South Sudan emergency. Available at: https://www.unhcr.org/south-sudan-emergency.html. Accessed December 18, 2018.
6. United Nations Office for the Coordination of Humanitarian Affairs. OCHA: South Sudan, Republic of. Available at: https://www.unocha.org/south-sudan. Accessed December 18, 2018.
7. Calam R. Public health implications and risks for children and families resettled after exposure to armed conflict and displacement. Scand J Public Health 2017;45(3):209–11.
8. Kaplan I, Stolk Y, Valibhoy M, et al. Cognitive assessment of refugee children: effects of trauma and new language acquisition. Transcult Psychiatry 2016;53(1):81–109.
9. Ataiants J, Cohen C, Riley AH, et al. Unaccompanied children at the united states border, a human rights crisis that can be addressed with policy change. J Immigr Minor Health 2018;20(4):1000–10. Available at: https://www.ncbi.nlm.nih.gov/pubmed/28391501 https://www.ncbi.nlm.nih.gov/pmc/PMC5805654/.
10. International Organization for Migration. Missing migrants project: tracking deaths along migratory routes 2018. Available at: https://missingmigrants.iom.int/region/mediterranean. Accessed December 18, 2018.
11. Green A. Fighting restricts access to health care in South Sudan. Lancet 2014;384(9950):1252.

12. Silbermann M, Daher M, Kebudi R, et al. Middle eastern conflicts: implications for refugee health in the European union and middle eastern host countries. J Glob Oncol 2016;2(6):422–30. Available at: https://www.ncbi.nlm.nih.gov/pubmed/ 28717729 https://www.ncbi.nlm.nih.gov/pmc/PMC5493250/.
13. United Nations High Commissioner for Refugees. UNHCR: Dadaab refugee complex. Available at: https://www.unhcr.org/ke/dadaab-refugee-complex. Accessed December 18, 2018.
14. United Nations High Commissioner for Refugees. UNHCR: Kakuma refugee camp and Kalobeyei integrated settlement. Available at: https://www.unhcr.org/ ke/kakuma-refugee-camp. Accessed December 18, 2018.
15. World Health Organization. WHO health cluster current partners 2018. Available at: https://www.who.int/health-cluster/partners/current-partners/en/. Accessed December 18, 2018.
16. Peyrassol S, editor. The priorities – check-lists, indicators, standards – situation with displacement of population. 4th edition. Brussels (Belgium): Medecins Sans Frontieres; 2011.

Clinical Tools Working at Home with Immigrants and Refugees

Chloe Turner, MD[a,b], Anisa Ibrahim, MD[c], Julie M. Linton, MD[d,e],*

KEYWORDS

- Immigrant children • Medical home • Health literacy • Developmental screening
- Mental health screening • Social determinants of health

KEY POINTS

- As immigrant and refugee children enter care, pediatric providers can incorporate the following 6 domains for clinical care: setting the stage, creating a culturally safe and effective space, medical screening, developmental/learning assessment, mental health screening, and social determinants of health screening.
- As a fundamental concept to be integrated across the 6 domains for clinical care, an emphasis on health literacy should be incorporated throughout the clinical care of immigrant children.
- Pediatric providers should engage in efforts to build relationships with community-based organizations that can meet the needs of families in an effort to support optimal health and well-being.

INTRODUCTION

When all children can achieve optimal health, our communities benefit through enhanced public health, well-being, and collective prosperity. The proportion of children in immigrant families, defined as children who were born outside of the United States or have at least 1 parent who was born outside of the United States, continues to increase. In fact, 1 in 4 children in the United States live in immigrant families.[1,2] However, the population of immigrant children, defined as children who are foreign born, decreased by 21% (from 2.7 million to 2.1 million) between 2000 and 2016.[1]

Disclosure statement: None of the authors have conflicts of interest relevant to the work described.
[a] Unity Health Care, Inc., 3020 14th Street Northwest, Washington, DC 20009, USA; [b] A.T. Still University of Health Sciences, Mesa, AZ, USA; [c] Department of Pediatrics, University of Washington, Harborview Medical Center, 325 9th Avenue Box 359774, Seattle, WA 98104, USA; [d] University of South Carolina School of Medicine Greenville, Prisma Health Upstate Children's Hospital, 20 Medical Ridge Drive, Greenville, SC 29605, USA; [e] Wake Forest School of Medicine, Winston-Salem, NC, USA
* Corresponding author. Center for Pediatric Medicine, 20 Medical Ridge Drive, Greenville, SC 29605.
E-mail address: jlinton@ghs.org

At a time of evolving demographics and turbulent policy changes, pediatric providers have a critical role in the care of all children, regardless of where the child or parent was born.

Immigrant children have incredible strengths and unique needs that can be reinforced and addressed by pediatric providers. Access to comprehensive, high-quality care can support the health and well-being of immigrant children toward an overarching vision of health equity. Recognizing the impact of the family language preference, health insurance status, and family immigration status on access to and quality of care is essential when providing comprehensive care to immigrant children. Ongoing stressors for immigrant families may include actual or threatened family separation, housing insecurity, food insecurity, and compound trauma.[3–7] Protective factors may include family commitment and social cohesion.[8–10]

Pediatric providers can facilitate access to high-quality care and critical community-based resources for immigrant children and families. In this article, we intend to explain health literacy as a fundamental concept to emphasize throughout clinical care, delineate 6 primary domains for clinical care, and offer clinical tools to achieve provision of accessible, comprehensive, high quality care within a family-centered medical home.

HEALTH LITERACY

Navigating complex health care systems can be particularly daunting for immigrant families. who may experience language barriers, a limited understanding of health systems, the stress of resettlement, and isolation. Tasks that seem straightforward to the health care provider might indeed have multiple steps that are confusing to patients who have minimal knowledge regarding how to navigate a health care setting. The term health literacy, initially coined in the 1970s, is now defined as "the degree to which an individual has the capacity to obtain, communicate, process, and understand basic health information and services to make appropriate health decisions" by Title V of the 2010 Patient Protection and Affordable Care Act.[11] The term encompasses numerous skills that an individual must have to navigate and understand their health and health care. Health literacy includes educating patients about health topics and communicating in a language they understand. Health literacy is also grounded in the complex interactions between the patient and the physician that take into consideration a patient's cultural, education, and preferred language.

In 2003, 36% of the US adult population was found to have limited health literacy. Rates were higher for people who spoke another language before English, people living in poverty, and minorities.[12] Individuals with lower literacy levels have been shown to be 1.5 to 3.0 times more likely to experience negative health outcomes.[13] The impact of low health literacy can be far greater for immigrants who have additional barriers to health literacy including linguistic barriers, cultural barriers, and lack of familiarity of the health care system after the resettlement period.

Upon resettlement, immigrants often have a limited understanding of their host country's medical system and thus may face barriers in access to services, particularly preventive services. Although first-generation immigrants are often healthier than their nonimmigrant counterparts, this healthy migrant effect diminishes dramatically for a variety of reasons, including poverty, unhealthy lifestyle changes, and barriers to accessing health care.[14] In light of these expected challenges, particular care should be given to building health literacy in immigrant populations in the early resettlement period.

In many parts of the world, there is no framework for preventive care; therefore, the concept of seeking care without illness may not be established. Additionally, the concepts of a medical home and a primary care physician may be foreign. If families are able to initiate access to primary care, they may be lost in the matrix between their primary care physician, the dietician to whom they were referred for malnutrition, and the neurologist they see for seizures, for example. Parents may ask 1 physician a question that is not in their scope of practice and often have concerns left unaddressed because they are unsure which physician to approach next. Primary care providers and subspecialists are often not interconnected in a way that facilitates easy transfer of information, including family concerns, leaving families with low health literacy lost in this web. Owing to these challenges, new immigrants should receive an introduction to the health care system in their host country, ideally before or upon first contact with the health care system.

In the clinical setting, it may be difficult to ascertain an individual's health literacy without directly screening. Health literacy has been shown to increase with education. However, 44% of high school graduates and 12% of college graduates have below basic or basic health literacy levels.[15] For immigrants, these rates are compounded by limited language proficiency and cultural differences in accessing health care. Because health literacy cannot be accurately predicted based on education, other signs that emerge during interactions with patients may point to limited health literacy (**Box 1**).

If not addressed immediately, limited health literacy can have numerous consequences for the patients and families. A common example is a perceived lack of adherence to medication regimens that continue for several months (eg, iron supplementation, latent tuberculosis [TB] treatment). Patients are often instructed to pick up the first month's medication and then told that they have multiple refills. Unless refills are explained, patients may not understand that they have to present to the pharmacy to ask for another month's supply of medication to continue their treatment. This barrier is compounded by limited language services at many pharmacies. Patients then take only the first month of long-term medications and either wait multiple months until their next appointment to ask for more medications or assume that they have completed the treatment regimen. By understanding the obstacles patients face within an unfamiliar system, pediatric providers can begin to formulate interventions that lead to increased health literacy.

Interventions to address and promote health literacy must be multifaceted. "Universal precautions" for health literacy incorporate the notion that all patients may have difficulty comprehending health information and accessing services.[16] Effectively addressing low health literacy also requires that language and cultural barriers be addressed simultaneously.[17] Clear and concise communication with trained medical interpreters can aid in addressing language barriers in immigrant families. An awareness of how cultures learn new information is also vital. Eighty percent of the world's population lives in oral and visual cultures; therefore, learning occurs

---

Box 1
Red flags for limited health literacy

- Increased number of missed appointments
- Limited follow-through with plans and referrals
- Nonadherence with medications
- Incomplete forms
- Not asking questions during visits

through listening and watching.[18] Written materials, therefore, do not meaningfully reach immigrant communities who prefer to learn through oral traditions. This difference puts these families at a particular disadvantage. To address this difference, written instructions should be drafted in easy to understand terms and should be prefaced by a verbal explanation of the content with room to ask questions.

Improving health literacy extends beyond the medical encounter. Outside of the clinical setting, general adult and child literacy should be promoted and addressed. National campaigns such as the Reach Out and Read program promote early literacy in low-income settings.[19–21] Adult literacy and educational programs may vary by region, but should be supported both by policy and within communities because low literacy is a health disparity that will inevitably lead to poor health outcomes for the community.

KEY CLINICAL DOMAINS

According to the American Academy of Pediatrics, medical care of infants, children, and adolescents in a medical home should be accessible, continuous, comprehensive, family centered, coordinated, compassionate, and culturally effective.[22] As immigrant and refugee children enter care, providers can incorporate the following 6 domains into the provision of care in a medical home: setting the stage, creating a culturally safe and effective space, medical screening, developmental/learning assessment, mental health screening, and social determinants of health screening.

Setting the Stage in the Medical Home

The initial medical encounter for an immigrant child with a pediatric provider in a medical home can be instrumental in the development of a trusting doctor–patient partnership. Setting the stage for a clinical encounter with an immigrant child includes several key components. A welcoming introduction, including a description of roles of the medical team members, clinic logistics, and an explanation of what to expect during the visit, can help to set the stage for a mutually beneficial, productive, and rapport-building encounter. Pediatric providers should set aside time to explain the concept of preventive care. A newly arrived immigrant child may present on a pediatric provider's schedule without being identified before the visit. Recognizing that a child is a newly arrived immigrant can trigger unique considerations for the pediatric provider, making the identification of these patients critically important. Practices should consider instituting a standard way of asking if new patients are newly arrived to the country.

It is helpful for pediatric providers to explain that it is their duty and responsibility to ask sensitive questions with the purpose of fully understanding a child's health and best supporting the family. Families should be reassured that information shared in the health care setting is confidential and that pediatric providers are not involved with immigration enforcement.[6,23] Health care providers and patients have legal rights regarding shared information, and federal and state privacy laws provide protections to limit patient information disclosure (including immigration status-related data) to law enforcement officials.[24] However, pediatric providers need to make patients aware that certain situations and circumstances may create limitations to confidentiality, owing to legal reasons (situations in which the patient is at risk for serious/immediate physical harm, as in suicide, homicide, or abuse/neglect) and practical purposes (for communication to facilitate appropriate care coordination and treatment).[25]

Creating a Culturally Safe and Effective Space

Creating a safe, supportive space in the medical home involves providing culturally effective and linguistically appropriate health care services that serve to decrease health disparities.[26] Key concepts include cultural humility and cultural safety. Cultural humility incorporates "a lifelong commitment to self-evaluation and self-critique, to redressing the power imbalances in the patient-physician dynamic, and to developing mutually beneficial and nonpaternalistic clinical and advocacy partnerships with communities."[27] Cultural safety in medical education and practice encompasses a critical consideration of power relationships and patients' rights in health care, as well as a thorough regard for the physical, mental, social, spiritual, and cultural context of caring for a patient and community.[28] Culturally safe and effective spaces are further supported through familiarity with cultural values, ongoing cultural competency training for staff, and recruitment of staff members who reflect the community's diversity.[29]

Creating a culturally safe and effective space necessitates effective communication across language differences. Language barriers can result in less timely medical care, confusion, dissatisfaction, and medical errors; providing linguistically appropriate communication can serve to decrease these barriers.[30] Trained medical interpreters, including on-site interpreters, video services, or telephone interpreter services, decrease errors and improve communication with families who have limited English proficiency.[30,31] Given the potential for inadvertent interpretive errors, omissions, and editorializing sensitive information, it is best to avoid using untrained staff or family members, especially children.[6,30,31]

To support the best interaction and meaningful connection during a visit that uses interpreter services, pediatric providers should maintain eye contact with the child and/or family member (rather than the interpreter), speak clearly and slowly, prevent interruptions, avoid jargon, and pay attention to nonverbal cues and body language. It can be helpful to provide a brief summary to the interpreter at the beginning of the visit and debrief at the end. Providers should be mindful of offering language-appropriate forms and health education information materials to families.[32,33] For instance, when explaining concepts, use simple language (eg, say swallow instead of take pills) and ask questions to assess for understanding.[34] Providers who self-identify as proficient in a language other than English should undergo formal evaluation regarding their capacity to provide medical care in the identified language.[35,36]

Medical Evaluation

A comprehensive evaluation

A comprehensive medical evaluation for recently arrived immigrant and refugee children entails routinely recommended screening (based on age and risk factors), as well as considerations of the child or adolescent's unique experiences, circumstances, and background.[23,37,38] A comprehensive history, within the medical home, should include typical components with additional considerations, including unchecked or undiagnosed chronic medical illnesses (given the potential for lack of routine primary care in their home country), acute issues from journey to the United States, TB screening, consideration of other potential infectious diseases, catch-up immunizations, and dental care.[23,39] Key resources offer detailed information regarding comprehensive evaluation (**Table 1**).

Previous medical records and immunizations

Any medical records that the family or child may have (eg, medical and vaccine records from their country of origin and/or predeparture evaluations by panel physicians from the Centers for Disease Control and Prevention (CDC) overseas, screening tests,

Table 1
Key clinical tools for medical screening

Resource	Website
Centers for Disease Control and Prevention (CDC) Immigrant and Refugee Health Guidelines	https://www.cdc.gov/immigrantrefugeehealth/index.html
American Academy of Pediatrics (AAP) Immigrant Child Health Toolkit	https://www.aap.org/en-us/advocacy-and-policy/aap-health-initiatives/Immigrant-Child-Health-Toolkit/Pages/Immigrant-Child-Health-Toolkit.aspx
AAP Red Book: 2018 Report of the Committee on Infectious Diseases	https://redbook.solutions.aap.org/redbook.aspx
Centers for Disease Control and Prevention (CDC) Immunization Guidelines	https://www.cdc.gov/vaccines/schedules/index.html https://www.cdc.gov/vaccines/hcp/acip-recs/
DC AAP Immigrant Child Health Toolkit (an example of a user-friendly provider toolkit adapted with local resources)	http://aapdc.org/toolkit/immigranthealth/

laboratory results, treatment for parasitic infections, and evaluations and treatment while in Office of Refugee Resettlement custody) should be carefully reviewed, documented, and considered valid.[23] It is important to review immunization records if available, seek to obtain them if possible, and assess the need for catch-up immunizations depending on the child's age and previous vaccination status, per the CDC schedule and guidelines. If no records are available, vaccination or revaccination according to the CDC recommended catch-up vaccine schedule is the standard of care.[40] Pediatric providers may consider checking serologic tests, if feasible, available, and cost effective.[41]

History and physical examination
Taking a meaningful medical history for immigrant children is grounded in creating a trusting, sensitive environment and building rapport with a child and family. A detailed social history explores family structure, primary caregiver/legal guardian, social support, an understanding of who has played a role in caring for the child during their lives, and details about migration. Shifting family dynamics and family reunification or separation can influence children's well-being.[23] Details regarding immigration should not be documented in the medical record unless the pediatric provider is specifically working with an immigration lawyer who is representing the child or family.[24]

During a comprehensive examination, a leading priority is to identify undiagnosed or untreated conditions, given that many children many not have had access to routine medical care in their home country. Essential components include evaluation of growth parameters (weight, height, body mass index, and head circumference, as appropriate for age), nutrition status, blood pressure evaluation, vision screening, hearing evaluation for children over 4 years old or any child who did not have a newborn hearing screening, and a complete physical examination.[23,39] Dental evaluation is of high importance, given the prevalence of dental issues and potentially limited access to preventive dental care and treatment in countries of origin. Children should be referred to a dentist and educated about brushing teeth and avoiding sugary drinks and snacks.[23]

An evaluation of pubertal development includes assessing Tanner stage. Screening for female genital cutting in at-risk populations is recommended, recognizing the complex cultural values, norms, and sensitivities around this practice. There are clinics that are trained and experienced in assessing and communicating with families about issues with female genital cutting.[42]

Laboratory screening

Key resources can assist pediatric providers in identifying pertinent laboratory screening in immigrant and refugee children (see **Table 1**).[23,37,38] Recommended laboratory studies include general baseline screening as well as further screening and diagnostic studies to consider based on geography, exposures, and clinical presentation. For instance, a complete blood count with differential would be recommended for nearly all newly arrived immigrant children, in particular to screen for anemia and eosinophilia. However, screening (or presumptive treatment) for schistosomiasis may be considered for a child from sub-Saharan Africa. Similarly, screening for vitamin D deficiency may be considered for a child who wears a hijab and has limited sun exposure.

An evaluation for the signs and symptoms of TB, a history of contacts with TB, physical examination, and universal TB testing, regardless of history of Bacillus of Calmette and Guerin, should be done in all immigrant and refugee children. This can be done with tuberculin skin testing in children under age 2 or by interferon gamma release assay in children age 2 and older (including those with previous Bacillus of Calmette and Guerin vaccination). Positive results should prompt a chest radiograph to rule out active pulmonary TB, and treatment for latent TB should be considered as appropriate.[38]

Assessment of Development, Learning, and Participation in School

Refugee and immigrant children often have a disruption of the basic "scaffolding of childhood," or the basic experiences that are necessary for children to grow and thrive.[43] The immigration experience places children at increased risk for exposure to trauma, neglect, malnutrition, poor health, and a lack of educational opportunities. Each of these experiences in turn has an effect on their childhood development and their developmental trajectory. However, many children do not receive an adequate developmental assessment upon immigration.[44] Pediatric providers must consider the impact of specific challenges and obstacles on the development of immigrant children and incorporate screening and referral into clinical practice.

Discussing development with immigrant families first requires the pediatric provider to evaluate whether there is a cultural framework for the concept of development. In a 2016 study of developmental screening in refugee families, almost all participants reported that there is no word for development in their language, and many had limited knowledge of developmental milestones.[45] This limited awareness of milestones is compounded by cultural beliefs regarding developmental delays and societal stigmas that decrease a parent's desire to discuss their child's development or reveal their concerns. Parents reported being more concerned or more likely to raise concerns with a provider if there were speech or behavioral problems and less like to bring up concerns when children have a physical disability. Barriers to recognizing and discussing developmental delays in refugee and immigrant children include limited formal education, cultural factors that influence when a child is considered delayed, low health literacy, and language barriers. Despite numerous challenges, the use of routine developmental screening methods were supported (**Table 2**), and the screening questionnaire was found to be a useful avenue to teach families about developmental milestones and discuss norms.

A family-centered approach to developmental screening facilitates partnership with the parent(s) and the creation of a meaningful management plan, should the child be diagnosed with a delay. Furthermore, similar to developmental milestones, many

Table 2
Key developmental screening for immigrant children

Resource	Website
Parents' Evaluation of Developmental Status (PEDS)	http://www.pedstest.com/default.aspx
Ages and Stages Questionnaire (ASQ)	https://agesandstages.com/
Ages and Stages Questionnaire: Social and Emotional (ASQ-SE)	http://www.brookespublishing.com/resource-center/screening-and-assessment/asq/asq-se-2/
Modified Checklist for Autism in Toddlers (M-CHAT)	https://www.m-chat.org/index.php
Survey of Well Being of Children (SWYC)	http://www.theswyc.org
US DHHS Birth to 5 Watch Me Thrive	https://www.acf.hhs.gov/ecd/child-health-development/watch-me-thrive

immigrants have no cultural framework for early intervention services, including therapy. A lack of familiarity with these services can translate into families being uncertain about the benefits. In the setting of positive screening or developmental concerns, key referrals are essential (**Table 3**). Engaging family educators or community health workers may facilitate successful developmental referrals.[46]

Table 3
Resources to support development and education

Resource	Website
Referrals for concerns for developmental delay	
Early intervention (ages 0–3 y)	State-based programs: https://www.cdc.gov/ncbddd/actearly/parents/states.html
Early intervention (age ≥3 y)	Contact local school system, Child Find: http://www.parentcenterhub.org/preschoolers/
Referrals that promote school readiness	
Reach Out and Read	http://www.reachoutandread.org/
Early Head Start (ages 0–3 y)	https://eclkc.ohs.acf.hhs.gov/programs/article/about-early-head-start-program
Head Start (ages 3–5 y)	https://www.acf.hhs.gov/ohs
Resources to support newly arrived families in schools	
Language support in schools	https://www2.ed.gov/about/offices/list/ocr/ellresources.html
Educational assessment	IDEA and Individualized Education Plan (IEP): https://sites.ed.gov/idea/statute-chapter-33/subchapter-II/1414 IDEA and Section 504: https://www2.ed.gov/about/offices/list/ocr/504faq.html?exp
Medical–legal partnership	Resource for parents or students whose educational needs are not being met: https://medical-legalpartnership.org/
After school programs and clubs	Varies by location, examples include: Boys and Girls Club https://www.bgca.org YMCA http://www.ymca.net/index.php Big Brother Big Sister https://www.bbbs.org Afterschool Programs https://youth.gov/youth-topics/afterschool-programs

Early childhood education

Early childhood education and care has become a norm in the United States and supports long-term health outcomes and well-being.[47] In 2005%, 73% of 2-year-old children in the United States had at least 1 weekly nonparental care arrangement.[48] Despite this rate, children of immigrants were less likely to be enrolled in preschool programs.[49] Although having an immigrant mother predicts a lower likelihood of nonparental care in the 0- to 2-year-old age group (controlling for other factors including socioeconomic status), immigrant children in the 3- to 5-year age groups had similar predictors of enrollment in early childhood education as nonimmigrant children. This finding demonstrates that underenrollment in early childhood education is not simply due to immigration status, but is multifactorial and involves maternal level of education and employment status. Early childhood education has been proven to decrease gaps in school readiness. However, increasing enrollment relies more on addressing inequities in socioeconomic status rather than immigration status.[50] Pediatric providers can familiarize themselves with local and national resources that support school readiness (see **Table 3**).

School

In the United States, every child has the right to a free, public education,[51] and attendance is expected. Furthermore, children with disabilities have the right to access appropriate public education.[52] However, this is not the experience of immigrant and refugee children globally. In 2011, there were 57 million children who were out of school globally; more than one-half of these children were in conflict-affected settings.[53] Once children resettle or immigrate, the success of their educational experience depends on their school and teachers' understanding of their prior educational experiences or lack thereof. Pediatric providers should inform families about their educational rights and empower them to advocate on behalf of children.

Four key themes illustrate the educational experience for refugee children in the country of first asylum, including limited and interrupted education, language barriers that limit access to education, poor quality or inadequate instruction, and discrimination in school settings.[54] When education is received, the instruction is often teacher centered and lecture based, creating a system where memorization, instead of active participation and problem solving, is valued. The conflicts that create these educational circumstances are unfortunately not short lived and often span the entire duration of a child's formal education. Children who are not formally considered refugees but immigrated often also face similar circumstances. Unfortunately, educational challenges do not end for these children once they are in their new communities. They must learn to adapt to their new home, culture, and education.

Developmental processes that are important for immigrant children include acculturation, ethnic identity formation, and bilingualism.[44] Acculturation, formally thought of as a unilateral process, is now seen as a bilateral process where immigrants also affect the communities where they resettle. Children rapidly socialize in school and quickly pick up the host culture, whereas parents do not have the same opportunities for socialization. This discrepancy leads to acculturation gaps within families, where children associate more with their host culture and parents aim for a balance of the 2 cultures. During this acculturation process, children, especially adolescents, often question their cultural identity. Although a strong ethnic identity is shown to be protective for immigrant adolescents, youth also strive to assimilate with their new environment's culture.[44] Children are more likely to be more successful in settings where their cultural identities are supported.

Language proficiency is central to immigrant children's success, both within and outside of the classroom. Immigrant and refugee children begin school with varying levels of English language proficiency. Without detailed assessments of their educational skills, they are often placed in classroom settings that are not congruent with their skill set. Furthermore, students may have a different understanding of expectations in the classroom setting as they move from a teacher-centered teaching style to child-centered instruction.[54] Students who may seem disengaged may actually be following that they believe is expected behavior in the classroom. Knowledge of a child's past educational experience, appropriate language support, and inclusivity in the school setting are important factors in supporting the success of immigrant children in the US educational system. Pediatric providers can incorporate this knowledge to inform and advocate for the children and their families and to connect children with resources available to them in the school system and in the community (see **Table 3**).

Mental Health Screening

The mental health of immigrant and refugee children is influenced by the context of their individual experiences in their country of origin, throughout their journey to the United States, and during resettlement after arrival. A trauma-informed, sensitive, and collaborative approach to working with vulnerable children and adolescents is vital in creating a safe space to explore stressors, screen for trauma, and connect families to mental and behavior health support resources.[55,56]

Experiences of stress may be related to trauma before leaving their home country (eg, as witnesses or victims of threats or violence, natural disasters, poverty, and attachment ruptures related to the disruption of family composition). During the migration journey, children may endure hazardous travel conditions, physical injuries, infections, diseases, exploitation and abuse, violence, sexual assault, detention at the border, and family separation. After arrival in the United States, children may experience discrimination, fear of deportation for family members or themselves, acculturative stress, language and cultural barriers, bullying at school, negative messages in the media related to race and immigration status, adjustment to a new social support structure, academic stressors, housing and food insecurity, and limited access to mental health support resources.[3,57] Throughout the migration journey, families may be apart for longer than anticipated for a variety of reasons, including economic needs, legal barriers, and immigration enforcement. Upon reunification, children may be placed in the care of family members in the United States who they have never met before or have not seen for years. Pediatric providers should be aware of a child's changing support structures, understand that the reunification process can be challenging, and work to promote positive family reunions and connect families to local and national support resources.[58,59]

Significant stress related to migration experiences and acculturation may manifest as mental health and behavior issues, which can have diverse presentations at distinctive ages and stages of development in children.[60] Toxic stress and adverse childhood experiences can adversely impact children's developing brain architecture and cause lifelong health effects. Toxic stress may manifest as changes in behavior and body function, which can include appetite or sleep disturbances, somatic complaints (such as frequent headaches or stomach pain), tantrums, regression (including regression of speech or toilet training in toddlers), attachment issues, aggression, and substance abuse. As a result of toxic stress, children may be at greater risk for post-traumatic stress disorder, depression, anxiety, and poor school performance.[3,57,61]

There is an expected adjustment period for any immigrant child, but when daily social, emotional, and academic functioning are impacted, intervention may be warranted.[57]

The American Academy of Pediatrics recommends psychosocial screening at every well-child visit with the goal of identifying children with mental health problems in a timely manner, intervening promptly, and providing support and treatment.[39] When evaluating trauma and mental health needs in immigrant and refugee children, it is important that pediatric providers pay respectful attention to cultural considerations and family engagement while assessing needs in the context of an individual's family, school, and community environment.[62,63] There are a variety of available mental health screening instruments and resources for immigrant and refugee children (**Table 4**).

Pediatric providers play a vital role in connecting families to mental and behavioral support resources, ideally colocated in the same setting as for other medical conditions, offering the opportunity to engage the family, decrease barriers to care, and access additional service coordination.[55,64,65] Resources include integrated behavioral health care, school-based services, and community-based mental health care.[66] For children with more complex mental health needs, child psychiatry access programs aim to connect primary care providers in the medical home with pediatric psychiatrists by phone consultation.[67] A multidisciplinary approach, involving medical personnel, social workers, teachers, school counselors, and immigration attorneys, can help to connect children to necessary services and support resilience in children and communities. Providing education on parenting and acculturative stress, offering linguistically appropriate and culturally relevant services, and fostering school engagement can help to bridge barriers to accessing medical and mental/behavioral health care for immigrant families. Gaining a familiarity with local and national resources can help pediatric providers to link families to necessary, culturally effective mental health providers and programs. Schools can serve as important places for integration of trauma-informed mental health prevention and treatment by decreasing barriers to access while also serving as a link with the local community for children and parents.[57] Trauma-focused counseling and interventions (for individuals or groups), including narrative exposure therapy for posttraumatic stress, trauma-focused cognitive–behavioral therapy for depression and anxiety, and family-oriented care models (including parent–child interaction therapy to enhance family functioning) may be effective interventions and can be school based.[68–70] Pediatric providers should also attend to the potential impact of secondary trauma on their own health and well-being.[71]

Table 4	
Key mental health screening tools for immigrant children	
Resource	**Website**
Strengths and Difficulties Questionnaire (SDQ)	http://www.sdqinfo.com/a0.html
Patient Health Questionnaire (PHQ-2/9)	https://www.phqscreeners.com/
Ages and Stages Questionnaire-Social Emotional (ASQ-SE)	http://agesandstages.com/products-services/asqse-2/
Survey of Wellbeing of Youth and Children (SWYC)	http://www.theswyc.org
Pediatric Symptom Checklist (17 or 35)	https://www.massgeneral.org/psychiatry/services/psc_home.aspx
Refugee Health Screener (RHS-15)	https://refugeehealthta.org/2012/02/08/refugee-health-screener-15-rhs-15/

Protective factors for immigrant children and families include interpersonal support and strong community connections.[23,72] Buffering relationships, particularly family and community support, offer a foundation for resilience. Pediatric providers can recognize potential adverse experiences that immigrant and refugee children may face, while also acknowledging unique strengths. Pediatric providers can play a vital role in fostering sources of supportive relationships in families, schools, and communities so as to increase protective factors, promote children's health, and help families to thrive.

Screening for Social Determinants of Health

Health care systems are increasingly acknowledging the role of the social determinants of health on provision of care and short- and long-term health outcomes. A number of screening tools and interventions exist to address the social determinants of health within pediatrics.[73–76] It is important to explore the needs of the community and understand the existing resources when selecting screening and intervention strategies.

Many social determinants of health that are relevant to all children (eg, poverty, food insecurity, housing insecurity, transportation, and formal education) may intersect with social determinants that are pronounced within immigrant families (eg, family immigration status and language preference). For instance, living in an immigrant family is itself a risk factor for food insecurity.[77] In the setting of heightened immigration enforcement, the risk of food insecurity among immigrant families may be intensified.[78] During a time of fear and uncertainty for immigrant families,[3] screening for social determinants of health may be particularly important.

When addressing social determinants of health, a unique consideration for immigrant families is legal need relating to immigration. Legal status often confers eligibility for public services, and medical documentation can support legal cases. However, in the clinical arena, most families will not self-identify as having legal needs relating to immigration. Thus, screening for legal needs can be particularly important. Some screening tools incorporate this into the screeners. Other programs may choose to adapt existing screeners to add a question such as, "Does your family need a lawyer to help with your landlord, housing, immigration, or taxes?" Before beginning and throughout implementation of screening, developing relationships with legal colleagues to make meaningful referral is critical to support immigrant families who may be facing threatened separation or are in removal proceedings. Additional research is needed to consider how to determine legal needs regarding immigration within the health care setting in a way that mitigates unintended harm (such as fear or reporting) and offers critical support to families.

Connecting families with local and national resources is a critical component of clinical care for all children. Within the medical home, integrated referral systems can be particularly helpful. For instance, medical–legal partnerships that incorporate immigration law can facilitate communication between medical and legal teams in an effort to improve legal outcomes.[79] In particular, warm hand-offs or in-person referrals that connect resources can limit potential breakdowns in communication.[80] Pediatric providers should engage in efforts to build relationships with community-based organizations that can meet the needs of families in an effort to support optimal health and well-being.

SUMMARY

The care of immigrant children should emphasize health literacy and incorporate a process to set the stage and screen for concerns regarding medical needs, development and education, mental health, and social determinants of health. Pediatric providers may consider a quality improvement process using Plan–Do–Study–Act cycles[81] to begin to incorporate the tools offered into the provision of care for immigrant children.

In a society where immigrant children face threats to their health and well-being coupled with opportunities to contribute immensely to our communities, pediatric providers play a critical role in building a foundation of equitable health care.

REFERENCES

1. Zong J, Batalova J, Hallock J. Frequently requested statistics on immigrants and immigration in the United States. Migration Information Source 2018. Available at: https://www.migrationpolicy.org/article/frequently-requested-statistics-immigrants-and-immigration-united-states. Accessed June 6, 2018.
2. Annie E. Casey foundation. Kids count data center 2018. Available at: http://datacenter.kidscount.org/. Accessed June 6, 2018.
3. Artiga S, Ubri P. Living in an immigrant family in America: how fear and toxic stress are affecting daily life, well-being, & health 2017. Available at: https://www.kff.org/disparities-policy/issue-brief/living-in-an-immigrant-family-in-america-how-fear-and-toxic-stress-are-affecting-daily-life-well-being-health/. Accessed March 14, 2019.
4. Perreira K, Ornelas I. Painful passages: traumatic experiences and post-traumatic stress among immigrant Latino adolescents and their primary caregivers. Int Migr Rev 2013;47(4). https://doi.org/10.1111/imre.12050.
5. Greenwald H, Zajfen V. Food insecurity and food resource utilization in an urban immigrant community. J Immigr Minor Health 2017;19(1):179–86.
6. Chilton L, Handal G, Paz-Soldan G. AAP council on community pediatrics. Providing care for immigrant, migrant, and border children. Pediatrics 2013;131(6):e2028–34.
7. Hernández D, Jiang Y, Carrión D, et al. Housing hardship and energy insecurity among native-born and immigrant low-income families with children in the United States. J Child Poverty 2016;22(2):77–92.
8. Denney J, Tolbert Kimbro R, Heck K, et al. Social cohesion and food insecurity: insights from the geographic research on wellbeing (GROW) study. Matern Child Health J 2017;21:343–50.
9. Perreira K, Marchante A, Schwartz S, et al. Stress and resilience: key correlates of mental health and substance use in the Hispanic community health study of Latino youth. J Immigr Minor Health 2019;21(1):4–13.
10. Landale N, Thomas K, Van Hook J. The living arrangements of children of immigrants. Future Child 2011;21(1):43–70.
11. Patient Protection and Affordable Care Act. 5 A U.S.C. § 5002 et seq.2010.
12. Berkman N, Sheridan S, Donahue K, et al. Health literacy interventions and outcomes: an updated systematic review. Evid Rep Technol Assess 2011;199:1–941.
13. DeWalt D, Berkman N, Sheridan S, et al. Literacy and health outcomes. J Gen Intern Med 2004;19(12):1228–39.
14. Zanchetta M, Poureslami I. Health literacy within the reality of immigrants' culture and language. Can J Public Health 2006;97(Suppl 2):S26–30.
15. U.S. Department of Health and Human Services. America's Health Literacy: why we need accessible health information. An issue brief from the U.S. Department

of Health and Human Services. Available at: https://health.gov/communication/literacy/issuebrief/. Accessed September 26, 2018.

16. AHRQ. AHRQ Health literacy universal precautions toolkit 2018. Available at: http://www.ahrq.gov/professionals/quality-patient-safety/quality-resources/tools/literacy-toolkit/index.html. Accessed September 5, 2018.

17. Shaw S, Huebner C, Armin J, et al. The role of culture in health literacy and chronic disease screening and management. J Immigr Minor Health 2009; 11(6):460–7.

18. Goody J. Literacy in traditional societies, vol. 19. Cambridge (United Kingdom): Cambridge University Press; 1968.

19. Sandler A. The impact of a clinic-based literacy intervention on language development in inner-city preschool children. J Dev Behav Pediatr 2001;22(4):265.

20. Sharif I, Rieber S, Ozuah P, et al. Exposure to reach out and read and vocabulary outcomes in inner city preschoolers. J Natl Med Assoc 2002;94(3):171–7.

21. Zuckerman B, Khandekar A. Reach out and read: evidence based approach to promoting early child development. Curr Opin Pediatr 2010;22(4):539–44.

22. American academy of pediatrics medical home initiatives for children with special needs project advisory committee. The medical home. Pediatrics 2002;110(1): 184–6.

23. American Academy of pediatrics Council on community pediatrics. Immigrant child health toolkit. 2015. Available at: https://www.aap.org/en-us/advocacy-and-policy/aap-health-initiatives/Immigrant-Child-Health-Toolkit/Pages/Immigrant-Child-Health-Toolkit.aspx. Accessed March 14, 2019.

24. National Immigration Law Center (NILC). Health care toolkits 2017. Available at: https://www.nilc.org/issues/immigration-enforcement/healthcare-provider-and-patients-rights-imm-enf/. Accessed July 30, 2018.

25. American Academy of Pediatrics Committee on child abuse and neglect. Child abuse. Confidentiality, and the health insurance portability and accountability act. Pediatrics 2010;125(1):197–201.

26. Brotanek J, Seeley C, Flores G. The importance of cultural competency in general pediatrics. Curr Opin Pediatr 2008;20(6):711–8.

27. Tervalon M, Murray-Garcia J. Cultural humility versus cultural competence: a critical distinction in defining physician training outcomes in multicultural education. J Health Care Poor Underserved 1998;9(2):117–25.

28. Papps P, Ramsden I. Cultural safety in nursing: the New Zealand experience. Int J Qual Health Care 1996;8(5):491–7.

29. Anderson L, Scrimshaw S, Fullilove MT, et al, Task Force on Community Preventive Services. Culturally competent healthcare systems: a systematic review. Am J Prev Med 2003;24(3 Supp):68–79.

30. Flores G, Laws M, Mayo S, et al. Errors in medical interpretation and their potential clinical consequences in pediatric encounters. Pediatrics 2003;111(1):6–14.

31. Jacobs B, Ryan A, Henrichs K, et al. Medical interpreters in outpatient practice. Ann Fam Med 2018;16(1):70–6.

32. U.S. Department of Health and Human Services Office of Minority Health. National standards for culturally and linguistically appropriate services in health care. Washington, DC: US Department of Health and Human Services Office of Minority Health; 2001.

33. American Academy of Pediatrics. AAP culturally effective care toolkit: engaging patients and families - interpretive services. Available at: https://www.aap.org/en-us/professional-resources/practice-transformation/managing-patients/Pages/chapter-5.aspx. Accessed August 5, 2018.

34. Federico F. 8 ways to improve health literacy 2014. Available at: http://www.ihi. org/communities/blogs/8-ways-to-improve-health-literacy. Accessed September 26, 2018.
35. National Council on Interpreting in Health care. What's in a word? A guide to understanding interpreting and translation in health care 2009. Available at: http://www.ncihc.org/assets/documents/publications/Whats_in_a_Word_Guide.pdf. Accessed March 14, 2019.
36. Kaiser Permanente and ALTA Language Services Inc. Clinician cultural and linguistic assessment (CCLA) 2018. Available at: https://www.altalang.com/language-testing/ccla/. Accessed August 8, 2018.
37. Centers for Disease Control and Prevention. Refugee health guidelines 2012. Available at: http://www.cdc.gov/immigrantrefugeehealth/guidelines/refugee-guidelines.html. Accessed July 30, 2018.
38. American Academy of Pediatrics. Red book: 2018 report of the committee on infectious diseases. In: Kimberlin D, Brady M, Jackson M, et al, editors. American academy of pediatrics. 2018. Available at: https://redbook.solutions.aap.org/redbook.aspx. Accessed March 14, 2019.
39. American Academy of Pediatrics. Bright futures: guidelines for health supervision of infants, children, and adolescents. 4th edition. Elk Grove Village (IL): American Academy of Pediatrics; 2017.
40. Centers for Disease Control and Prevention. Catch-up immunization schedule for persons aged 4 Months through 18 Years who start late or who are more than 1 Month behind 2018. Available at: https://www.cdc.gov/vaccines/schedules/hcp/imz/catchup.html. Accessed August 6, 2018.
41. US DHHS, Centers for Disease Control and Prevention. National center for emerging and zoonotic infectious diseases – division of global migration and quarantine. Guidelines for evaluating and updating immunizations during the domestic medical examination for newly arrived refugees 2015. Available at: https://www.cdc.gov/immigrantrefugeehealth/pdf/immunizations-guidelines.pdf. Accessed August 6, 2018.
42. Bridging Refugee Youth & Children's Services. Highlighted resources on female genital cutting 2018. Available at: http://www.brycs.org/clearinghouse/highlighted-resources-on-female-genital-cutting.cfm. Accessed August 6, 2018.
43. Refugee Health Technical Assistance Center. Youth and mental health 2018. Available at: https://refugeehealthta.org/refugee-basics/refugee-resettlement/. Accessed September 26, 2018.
44. Cowden J, Kreisler K. Development in children of immigrant families. Pediatr Clin North Am 2016;63(5):775–93.
45. Kroening A, Moore J, Welch T, et al. Developmental screening of refugees: a qualitative study. Pediatrics 2016;138(3):e20160234.
46. Linton J, Stockton M, Andrade B, et al. Integrating parenting support within and beyond the pediatric medical home. Glob Pediatr Health 2018;5. https://doi.org/10.1177/2333794X18769819.
47. Campbell F, Conti G, Heckman J, et al. Early childhood investments substantially boost adult health. Science 2014;343(6178):1478–85.
48. Iruka I, Carver P. Initial results from the 2005 NHES early childhood program participation survey (NCES 2006–075). Washington, DC: National Center for Education Statistics; 2006.
49. Magnuson K, Lahaie C, Waldfogel J. Preschool and school readiness of children of immigrants. Soc Sci Q 2006;87(5):1241–62.

50. Greenberg J, Kahn J. The influence of immigration status on early childhood education and care enrollment. J Early Child Res 2011;9(1):20–35.
51. United States Supreme Court. Plyler v. Doe. Vol. 80-15381982.
52. U.S. Department of Education. About IDEA 2018. Available at: https://sites.ed.gov/idea/about-idea/. Accessed September 26, 2018.
53. UNESCO. Children still battling to go to school. Paris: UNESCO; 2013.
54. Dryden-Peterson S. The educational experiences of refugee children in countries of first asylum. Washington, DC: Migration Policy Institute; 2015.
55. Caballero T, DeCamp L, Platt R, et al. Addressing the mental health needs of Latino children in immigrant families. Clin Pediatr 2017;56(7):648–58.
56. American Academy of Pediatrics. Trauma toolbox for primary care. In: Dowd MD, editor 2014. Available at: https://www.aap.org/en-us/advocacy-and-policy/aap-health-initiatives/healthy-foster-care-america/Pages/Trauma-Guide.aspx - trauma. Accessed July 30, 2016.
57. Fazel M, Stein A. The mental health of refugee children. Arch Dis Child 2002;87:366–70.
58. Fairfax county public schools. Immigrant Family Reunification Program; 2018. Available at: https://www.fcps.edu/resources/family-engagement/immigrant-family-reunification-program. Accessed August 6, 2018.
59. Fairfax County Public Schools, U.S. Committee for Refugees and Immigrants. Reconnecting families 2016. Fairfax (VA). Available at: http://refugees.org/wp-content/uploads/2016/03/Reconnecting-Families-Book-English.pdf. Accessed March 14, 2019.
60. Gonzales R, Suarez-Orozco C, Dedios-Sanguineti M. No place to belong: contextualizing concepts of mental health among undocumented immigrant youth in the United States. Am Behav Sci 2013;57:1174–99.
61. Garner AS, Shonkoff JP, Committee on Psychosocial Aspects of Child and Family Health; Committee on Early Childhood, Adoption, and Dependent Care; Section on Developmental and Behavioral Pediatrics. Early childhood adversity, toxic stress, and the role of the pediatrician: translating developmental science into lifelong health. Pediatrics 2012;129(1):e224–31.
62. The National Child Traumatic Stress Network. Refugee trauma: screening and assessment 2018. Available at: https://www.nctsn.org/what-is-child-trauma/trauma-types/refugee-trauma/screening-and-assessment. Accessed August 6, 2018.
63. Fazel M, Betancourt T. Preventive mental health interventions for refugee children and adolescents in high-income settings. Lancet Child Adolesc Health 2018;2:121–32.
64. Bridges A, Andrews A III, Villalobos B, et al. Does integrated behavioral health care reduce mental health disparities for Latinos? Initial findings. J Lat Pscyhol 2014;2(1):37–53.
65. Ader J, Stille C, Keller D, et al. The medical home and integrated behavior health: advancing the policy agenda. Pediatrics 2015;135(5):909–17.
66. Tyrer RA, Fazel M. School and community-based interventions for refugee and asylum seeking children: a systematic review. PloS One 2014;9(2):e89359.
67. National Network of Child Psychiatry Access Programs. Integrating mental and behavioral health care for every child 2018. Available at: http://www.nncpap.org. Accessed August 6, 2018.
68. Fazel M. Psychological and psychosocial interventions for refugee children resettled in high-income countries. Epidemiol Psychiatr Sci 2018;27(2):1170123.

69. Kataoka S, Stein B, Jaycox L, et al. A school-based mental health program for traumatized Latino immigrant children. J Am Acad Child Adolesc Psychiatry 2003;42(3):311–8.

70. Thordarson M, Keller M, Sullivan P, et al. Cognitive-behavioral therapy for immigrant youth: the essentials. In: Patel S, Reicherter D, editors. Psychotherapy for immigrant youth. Cham (Switzerland): Springer; 2016. p. 28–48.

71. National Child Traumatic Stress Network. Secondary traumatic stress: understanding who is at risk 2018. Available at: https://www.nctsn.org/trauma-informed-care/secondary-traumatic-stress/introduction. Accessed March 14, 2019.

72. Fazel M, Reed RV, Panter-Brick C, et al. Mental health of displaced and refugee children resettled in high-income countries: risk and protective factors. Lancet 2012;379(9812):266–82.

73. Garg A, Toy S, Tripodis Y, et al. Addressing social determinants of health at well child care visits: a cluster RCT. Pediatrics 2015;135(2):e296–304.

74. Kenyon C, Sandel M, Silverstein M, et al. Revisiting the social history for child health. Pediatrics 2007;120(3):e734–8.

75. Fazalullasha F, Taras J, Morinis J, et al. From office tools to community supports: the needs for infrastructure to address the social determinants of health in paediatric practice. Paediatr Child Health 2014;19(4):195–9.

76. Fierman A, Beck A, Chung E, et al. Redesigning health care practices to address childhood poverty. Acad Pediatr 2016;16:S136–46.

77. Chilton M, Black M, Berkowitz C, et al. Food insecurity and risk of poor health among US-born children of immigrants. Am J Public Health 2009;99(3):556–62.

78. Potochnick S, Chen J, Perreira K. Local-level immigration enforcement and food insecurity risk among Hispanic immigrant families with children: national-level evidence. J Immigr Minor Health 2017;19:1042–9.

79. Linton J, Kennedy E, Shapiro A, et al. Unaccompanied children seeking safe haven: providing care and supporting well-being of a vulnerable population. Child Youth Serv Rev 2018;92:122–32.

80. Agency for Healthcare Research and Quality (AHRQ). Design guide for implementing warm handoffs 2017. Available at: https://www.ahrq.gov/sites/default/files/wysiwyg/professionals/quality-patient-safety/patient-family-engagement/pfeprimarycare/warmhandoff-designguide.pdf. Accessed December 26, 2017.

81. Institute for Healthcare Improvement (IHI). Models for improvement 2018. Available at: http://www.ihi.org/resources/Pages/HowtoImprove/default.aspx. Accessed June 8, 2018.

Advocating for Immigration Policies that Promote Children's Health

Julie M. Linton, MD[a,b,*], Jennifer Nagda, JD[c],
Olanrewaju O. Falusi, MD[d]

KEYWORDS

• Immigrant children • Advocacy • Immigration policy • Social determinants of health

KEY POINTS

- Immigration status, like other social determinants of health, has a direct impact on children's access to health care, safe housing, food, and educational opportunities.
- Children who wish to remain permanently in the United States, or who are fighting to prevent their own deportation, are placed into a legal system designed for adults, where there are few special protections for children and where the few protections that exist could be eliminated by federal policy makers.
- Pediatricians, who witness first-hand how immigration policy affects the health of children in their practices, have a unique opportunity to advocate for policies that better protect the health of all children, including immigrant children.

INTRODUCTION

Immigration laws and policies have a direct and significant effect on the health and well-being of children and their families. The recent and near constant focus on immigration in the press and other public discourse has affected the lives of all children in the United States, whether they are immigrants themselves or live in immigrant families. One in 4 children in the United States lives in an immigrant family,[1] in which the child and/or at least one parent was foreign-born. Children in immigrant families reside in all 50 states (**Fig. 1**). At a time when immigration law and policies affect so

Disclosure Statement: The authors have no relevant conflicts of interest to disclose.
[a] University of South Carolina School of Medicine Greenville, Prisma Health Upstate Children's Hospital, 20 Medical Ridge Drive, Greenville, SC 29605, USA; [b] Wake Forest School of Medicine, Winston-Salem, NC, USA; [c] Young Center for Immigrant Children's Rights, 6020 South University Avenue, Chicago, IL 60637, USA; [d] George Washington University School of Medicine and Health Sciences, Children's National Health System, 2233 Wisconsin Avenue Northwest, Suite 317, Washington, DC 20007, USA
* Corresponding author. 20 Medical Ridge Drive, Greenville, SC 29605.
E-mail address: Julie.linton@prismahealth.org

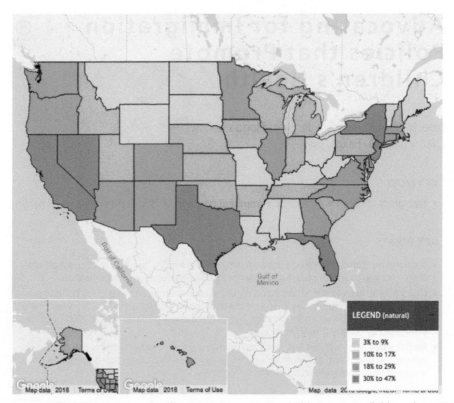

Fig. 1. Children in immigrant families, 2016. (*From* National Kids Count. Available at: https://datacenter.kidscount.org/. Accessed March 16, 2019. © 2008, The Annie E. Casey Foundation.)

many children, pediatricians have a particular responsibility to understand how those laws affect child health, and what they can do to advocate for immigration policies that promote better health for immigrant children.

Family migration often entails a complex spectrum of forced and voluntary components that, for some, includes the need for protection[1] and, for all, involves a search for a better future.[2] "Push factors" for migration may include humanitarian needs, such as natural disasters and armed conflict, which force people away from their countries of origin. "Pull factors" may include economic opportunities and educational aspirations,[3] as well as the prospect of reuniting with family.

A record of historically and currently inequitable immigration policy in the United States has made it increasingly difficult for families to successfully and safely immigrate to this nation. United States immigration policy has historically emphasized 3 key principles: family reunification for citizens and lawful permanent residents, admission of immigrants who offer skills that contribute to the United States economy, and humanitarian protection.[4] Although national-origins quotas were eliminated by the Immigration and Nationality Act of 1965, structural inequities in immigration enforcement continue to differentially affect populations.[5]

Recent policy changes, focused on limiting migration,[6] have worsened circumstances for immigrants coming to or living in the United States. Previous studies have shown that restrictive immigration policies have been associated with a negative impact on health and well-being.[7–10] Amid new policy changes, immigrant families have reported increased fear, uncertainty, and discrimination, regardless of immigration status.[11] Toxic stress, or serious prolonged stress in the absence of buffering support, adversely affects brain development and health of children.[12] Increased immigration enforcement has become a public health threat that health care professionals will inevitably face within practice and at the level of populations.

Understanding the complex reasons for migration and the journey that families experience can inform advocacy efforts that support the health and well-being of children and their families as they transition to life in the United States. The purpose of this article is to identify the impact of family immigration status and immigration laws on children's health, to understand the legal system faced by immigrant children, and to describe opportunities for health care professionals to engage in advocacy at the systems level, from the local community to the Hill.

FAMILY IMMIGRATION STATUS AS A SOCIAL DETERMINANT OF HEALTH

Family immigration status is a well-documented social determinant of health that contributes to health disparities. Social determinants of health (SDH or SDOH) are defined by Healthy People 2020 as "conditions in the environments in which people are born, live, learn, work, play, worship, and age that affect a wide range of health, functioning, and quality-of-life outcomes and risks."[13] SDH can become facilitators of, or barriers to, health equity, which is further defined by Healthy People 2020 as the "attainment of the highest level of health for all people."[14] Achieving health equity within the immigrant population requires a coordinated societal effort to address SDH and to correct discriminatory policies and practices. To effectively advocate for health equity for immigrant children and families, it is critical to recognize how immigration status intersects with a number of social factors to affect the health, well-being, and self-actualization—and that fear of immigration enforcement may hinder immigrant families from accessing programs that address social determinants. Although these social determinants are described separately in this article, it is clear that they are interconnected and can have additive effects.

Access to Health Care

Immigrant children without legal status are nearly 5 times as likely to be uninsured than children who are United States citizens. Having legal status does not eliminate the disparity in insurance status because lawfully present immigrant children are still 3 times as likely to be uninsured than United States citizens.[15] Most immigrant adults must wait 5 years after obtaining lawful permanent residence (also known as "green card" status) before they can qualify for Medicaid. Over half of the states have chosen to waive the 5-year wait for children and pregnant women. Immigrants without permanent legal status are not eligible for most federal programs or for subsidies under the Affordable Care Act, contributing to the wide gaps in coverage for this population. A few jurisdictions use local funds to expand Medicaid to cover all income-eligible children regardless of immigration status (**Fig. 2**).[16]

Having health insurance is associated with a reduction in health disparities and improvement in health outcomes. However, health insurance alone does not guarantee better health, and children in immigrant families may face further barriers to accessing health care. For example, Hispanic children with insurance, compared with insured non-Hispanic black and non-Hispanic white children, are the least likely

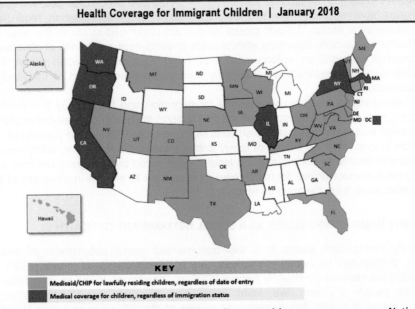

Fig. 2. Health coverage for immigrant children. (*From* Health care coverage maps. National Immigration Law Center, 2018. Available at: https://www.nilc.org/issues/health-care/healthcoveragemaps/. Accessed September 7, 2018.)

to have a usual source of health care and to use health care services, especially preventive services.[17,18] Decreased access to care manifests as immigrant children having higher rates of untreated stress, trauma, and depression[19] and twice the prevalence of early childhood caries.[20]

Poverty

Immigrants are generally more likely to live in poverty than the native-born population, with rates of 13.1% and 12.3%, respectively. The trend holds among immigrant children specifically, with first-generation immigrant children having a poverty rate 50% higher than native-born children. Compared with their peers, children living in poverty are more likely to have health problems such as low birth weight, lead poisoning, and behavioral and emotional problems. Children living in poverty are also more likely to be exposed to violence and suffer from injury and chronic illnesses.[21]

The higher rates of poverty among immigrant families persist despite immigrant children being more likely to live in 2-parent households and more than 90% of immigrant children having a parent who works. There are wide variations within the immigrant population, however, with foreign-born naturalized citizens experiencing a lower rate of poverty than native-born citizens (10.0% vs 12.3%), while nearly 20% of noncitizens live in poverty.[22] There is also variation based on race, as black immigrant families are less likely to live in poverty and are more likely to have higher education than native-born black families.[23] The reasons for the higher poverty rate among immigrants are multifaceted and include low-wage employment (including lower than minimum wage in some industries that hire undocumented workers) and living in larger families.[19]

Food Insecurity and Access to Public Services

Food insecurity, the "household-level economic and social condition of limited or uncertain access to adequate food,"[24] places children at higher risk of iron deficiency, dysregulated behavior, lower academic achievement, and other adverse sequelae.[25] The US Department of Agriculture, which monitors food insecurity rates based on race/ethnicity though not specifically immigrant status, has found that 11.6% of Hispanic households with children experienced food insecurity at some point in 2016, compared with 8% across all households with children.[24] Children of immigrants are more likely to experience food insecurity than are children of United States citizens, with children of parents without legal status and newly arrived immigrants at highest risk.[26–29] Fear of immigration enforcement may inhibit immigrant families from accessing programs such as the Supplemental Nutrition Assistance Program (SNAP, formerly food stamps) and the Women, Infants, and Children Program, even if the parent or the child is eligible.

Although families without legal status may be at higher risk of food insecurity than immigrant families with legal status, recent federal actions regarding the public charge definition may put all immigrant families in the United States at greater risk of food insecurity, poverty, and even deportation. For decades, the United States government has denied entry to the United States—or denied change of status to legal permanent residency for those already in the United States—to those deemed a likely public charge, or someone who would become financially dependent on the government. Traditionally the scope has been narrow, with a potential public charge defined as an individual who had used cash benefits or long-term institutionalization with federal funding. However, materials from the Department of Homeland Security (DHS) released in 2018 have caused great concern in immigrant communities and those who advocate for them. The expectation is that the public charge definition will broaden widely to include several noncash benefits, such as Medicaid, SNAP, and housing assistance. The Migration Policy Institute estimates that nearly half of immigrant families would fall under this new definition, compared with only 3% with the traditional definition.[30]

The significance of the public charge determination to children and food insecurity cannot be understated. Beyond the direct effect on certain immigrant families, the "chilling effect" of this change in policy has already been noted widely, with pediatricians around the country reporting families disenrolling their children from federal programs, or choosing not to enroll newborns in food assistance programs.[15,30] As of this writing the DHS regulation has not yet been implemented, but it is clear that the negative public health effect has already begun. Because eligibility for federal and state programs is complex, pediatricians are encouraged to familiarize themselves with eligibility criteria for programs in their community to facilitate patient access while also being aware about whether the use of such programs could affect future immigration status such as through a public charge determination.

Education

Children's right to an education stands in stark contrast to the right to access health services. In 1982, the Supreme Court found that all children, regardless of immigration status, have the right to a free and public education. In reaching this decision, the court found that denying children access to school because of their immigration status, a factor beyond their ability to control, would deny them the equal protections guaranteed to them by the Constitution.[31,32] Immigrant parents and students with limited English proficiency are also entitled to language-assistance services, including English-learning classes for students, report cards and parent handbooks in their preferred language, and interpreters at parent-teacher conferences at no cost to the parent. Secondary services, such as transportation, school-based health services, and free or reduced meals, must also be available regardless of a student's immigration status.[33] Several jurisdictions have attempted to circumvent this constitutional right to educational equity by collecting and reporting data on students' immigration status, requiring Social Security numbers on school registration, or outright prohibition of admitting students without lawful status.[34] Each of these measures was struck down by local and federal efforts. Protecting the rights of immigrant children to free public K-12 education is vital, as higher educational level has been associated with better health and longer life expectancy.[35,36]

Racial/Ethnic Discrimination and Stereotyping

Racial/ethnic discrimination is common among immigrant children and adults, with more than 70% of racial minority (ie, non-white) immigrants reporting having ever experienced discrimination, compared with less than 30% of their white counterparts.[37,38] This discrimination can manifest overtly, such as receiving poor service in stores and restaurants, being called offensive names, or being threatened or harassed; or more subtly, such as being treated with less courtesy and less respect, people acting as if they were not as smart as others, or people acting as if they were better than them.[37,39] Latino and black Caribbean immigrants are more likely to report everyday discrimination if they are male, younger, unmarried, more educated, earning higher incomes, or have lived in the United States for longer duration, suggesting that increased exposure to the majority population increases the risk of experiencing discrimination.[37–39]

Among adolescents, racial discrimination is negatively associated with civic beliefs. In one study, immigrant adolescents who reported experiencing racial discrimination were less likely to trust in the United States government or to believe that the government is responsive to individuals like them. This is relevant in the long term because trust in the responsiveness of government is a key marker of civic contribution, leading to better integration in the host country.[40] In addition, discrimination can have negative effects on physical and psychological well-being, including an increase in depressive symptoms and post-traumatic stress, and a decrease in self-esteem among various immigrant and ethnic minority communities.[41,42] Consequently, adolescents in one study who experienced greater post-traumatic stress symptoms reported more alcohol use and other drug use, involvement in more fights, and more sexual partners.[41] In another study, experiencing racism decreased the academic performance of foreign-born students.[43] The effects of positive stereotyping can also negatively affect the health of immigrant youth. For example, the model minority stereotype has been shown to contribute to Asian American youth's pressure to perform academically and occupationally at a level that seems unattainable. There may also be a lack of recognition of mental health concerns (eg, depression, suicidal ideation) in these communities.[43]

Housing Inequity

The location of one's home determines the availability of quality public education, grocery stores, neighborhood safety, and socialization within and across cultures. Inadequate housing conditions can increase the risk of asthma exacerbations, lead poisoning, and mental illness.[44,45] Immigrant families experience insufficient or crowded housing at disproportionately high rates.[46,47] Affordability of adequate housing and discrimination in renting and buying practices hamper the ability of immigrant families, particularly those in poverty, to ensure a home and neighborhood supportive of children's health and development.

In the face of these adversities, there are mitigating factors about which clinicians should be aware. Time spent in nature has been shown to reduce stress and improve physical health.[48,49] Moreover, immigrant families have described time spent in nature as an opportunity for their children to move freely and explore, thereby promoting their development and socialization with others.[50] Families experiencing discrimination have recourse through the Fair Housing Act, Title VIII of the Civil Rights Act of 1968, which prohibits housing discrimination for reasons including (but not limited to) race, color, and national origin.[51] It is illegal to retaliate against a complaint (for a landlord to threaten to call immigration enforcement after a renter submits a complaint about unfair leasing practices, for example), but this fear of retaliation leading to homelessness or deportation is pervasive in immigrant communities.

THE LEGAL SYSTEM GOVERNING THE RIGHTS OF CHILDREN TO SEEK PROTECTION OR REMAIN PERMANENTLY IN THE UNITED STATES

This section provides an overview of the legal system faced by children when they are placed into immigration removal (deportation) proceedings and the lack of child-specific protections that undermine children's safety, well-being, and permanency; the limited options for children who wish to remain permanently in the United States; and recent changes in federal immigration policy that further threaten children's safety and well-being.

Children in Immigration Proceedings

In this article, we use the term "immigration proceedings" as a shorthand for the wide range of processes whereby immigrant children, like adults, can be returned to their countries of origin or receive permission to remain temporarily or permanently in the United States. Immigration proceedings may occur in a formal courtroom before an immigration judge, in an interview setting with a government official, through a paper-based application, or via a combination of all 3. Similarly, the types of children subjected to these immigration proceedings have a range of backgrounds. The way in which they arrive in the country, the people with whom they arrive, and the location of their arrival—or the location of their discovery by immigration officials—all affect how their cases will be adjudicated.

Unaccompanied children

Many of the procedures described in the remainder of this section were developed for a specific group of children, known in the law as "unaccompanied alien children" (hereafter "unaccompanied immigrant children"). Immigration officials who encounter children must designate them as unaccompanied if they are: (1) younger than age of 18 years; (2) do not have lawful immigration status; and (3) for whom there is no parent or legal guardian in the United States or for whom there is no parent or legal guardian available to provide care or physical custody.[24] The last element of the definition can be confusing: most unaccompanied immigrant children are encountered at the border, arriving without a parent or legal guardian. However, they may have come with the hope of reunifying with a parent, family member, or friend in the United States, or they may be fleeing an abusive parent in their home country (or both). Children may also be designated as unaccompanied when found far away from the border, living in the United States—for example, when immigration officials conduct a raid, encounter a child, and there is no parent or legal guardian available to take custody of the child. When immigration officials encounter an unaccompanied immigrant child, they must transfer the child to the physical custody of the Office of Refugee Resettlement (ORR) within the Department of Health and Human Services (HHS) within 72 hours.[25] In general, unaccompanied immigrant children are placed into formal removal (deportation) proceedings before an immigration judge where, as described hereafter, they face the charge of being in the country without permission and carry the burden to prove their eligibility to remain.

Accompanied children

Children who arrive at the border *with* their parents are considered "accompanied" and are generally processed side by side with their parents; this puts them in a significantly different position from their unaccompanied counterparts. Adults and families apprehended at the border are typically subject to "expedited removal" proceedings, which means they may never have the opportunity to appear in front of an immigration judge. Rather, they are interviewed shortly after their apprehension and will be deported unless they can prove that they have a "credible fear of return"—a complicated legal standard. If they meet the "credible fear" test, they will have the opportunity to proceed with a full case before an immigration judge. In recent years, as the number of families arriving at the border has increased, the government has responded by detaining, rather than immediately releasing, many families as they work through this multistep legal process.[24] In response, advocates for children and families have fought to limit the time children spend in these family detention facilities, to change the conditions within the facilities, and to protest the use of and licensing of these facilities.[26]

Notably, in 2018 the government launched a policy to forcibly separate accompanied children from their parents at the border to prosecute parents for entering the United States without permission or for re-entering after a prior deportation.[27] As described later, this effort was part of a larger effort to deter the migration of families from Central America. As a result of the policy, thousands of children were rendered unaccompanied by immigration officials.[28] After significant public outcry and litigation by the American Civil Liberties Union and children's advocates, many separated families were reunited[29] but the status of both the parents' and children's legal cases remain in limbo, at best, at the time of publication.

Children living within the United States

Finally, children living within the United State who lack legal status but who have not encountered immigration authorities may decide to affirmatively present themselves to immigration authorities to apply for some of the protections discussed hereafter, such as asylum, Special Immigrant Juvenile Status (SIJS), or "T" or "U" nonimmigrant status. They may do this in coordination with parents, as part of a parent's application for a benefit, or completely independent of parents and family members.

Lack of Protections that Undermine Children's Safety, Well-Being, and Permanency

Immigration proceedings were not designed for children and lack many of the protections extended to children in other legal proceedings. This article cannot comprehensively address the system of adjudicating children's immigration cases but instead focuses on 3 features of the immigration system that significantly limit children's ability to access fair proceedings that would better ensure their safety and well-being.

Adversarial proceedings
Children who are discovered by or present themselves to immigration authorities are generally charged with being in the country without permission and placed into formal immigration proceedings, known as removal proceedings.[a] These proceedings are adversarial in nature: the government is the "Petitioner" and is represented by an attorney who argues for the child's removal from the country. The child is the "Respondent" and carries the burden of proving her case. The decision of whether the child may remain in the United States or must return is made by an immigration judge. Cases are heard in formal courtrooms, where the judge sits on a dais wearing a robe. Children can be cross-examined by the government attorney. If the government attorney can identify factual inconsistencies in the child's story, the immigration judge may determine that the child lacks credibility and deny the child's claim for protection, notwithstanding the impact of age, trauma, or other factors on the child's ability to testify or consistently recount his or her story.

No explicit "best interests of the child" mandate for key decisions
The best interests of the child standard—the hallmark of child protection proceedings in state court—appears in immigration law only sparingly.[30] The ORR, which takes custody of unaccompanied children, is required to place immigrant children in the least restrictive setting that is in their best interests.[52] In 2008, Congress authorized the federal government to appoint independent Child Advocates to identify and advocate for the best interests of unaccompanied children and child trafficking victims.[53] Over the years, agencies and decision-makers have relied on Child Advocates' recommendations when making decisions about the most vulnerable children to whom Child Advocates are appointed,[54] but there is no specific mandate under immigration law that requires every actor to consider the best interests of each immigrant child in every decision. Thus, there is no requirement to consider a child's best interests in some of the most important decisions made by immigration officials, such as: deciding whether to separate a child from family at the border; whether to grant a child more time to find a lawyer; whether to grant a child asylum or lawful permanent residence; or whether to order a child returned to his or her country of origin.

No attorney at government expense
Individuals in immigration proceedings are entitled to be represented by attorneys but not at government expense.[55] More specifically, the government is not obligated to provide lawyers to children who cannot find or afford their own attorney, despite the consequences of immigration proceedings, which can include prolonged detention, separation from family, and deportation. Compare this with children in delinquency proceedings, who for 50 years have had the constitutional right to representation by counsel.[56] Children in immigration proceedings arguably face stakes equal to those of youth in delinquency proceedings or adults in criminal proceedings, including restrictions on liberty and the possibility of deportation. However, recent challenges to win the same right to counsel for immigrant children have not yet succeeded.[57]

---

[a] Children apprehended at the border with a parent are generally placed in special proceedings with that parent, known as expedited removal. In expedited removal proceedings, parents and children appear in front of an asylum officer rather than an immigration judge. Unless the parent and children can demonstrate that they have a "credible fear" of return to their country, they will be removed (deported) without an opportunity to appear before a judge. Parents (and children) who do establish "credible fear" will then have an opportunity to appear in front of a judge and raise as many defenses to removal (deportation) as possible.

The Difficult and Limited Options Faced by Children if They Wish to Remain in the United States

In general, children who do not have lawful immigration status and who wish to remain in the United States must apply for the very same forms of protection from removal that were established for adults. With one exception (SIJS, **Table 1**), there are no forms of protection that are specific to children. Although there are some special procedures for children, in general their cases proceed on the same path and in the same places as adults' cases. **Table 1** provides an intentionally general overview of these forms of protection—they are not comprehensive and should not be used to determine whether any specific person might be eligible to apply for protection.

Recent Changes in Federal Immigration Policy

Immigrant children and families stand on the front line of the current battle over immigration policy.[b] Since January 2017, the Executive Branch has sought to deter or limit migration to the United States through a range of policy changes, many targeting children and their families. Moreover, the rhetoric accompanying these changes often targets children as threats or as loophole exploiters. These changes in policy and the accompanying rhetoric negatively affect children's sense of safety, security, and permanency.

The disruption of family integrity has been a core component of the Trump Administration's efforts to deter migration and change immigration policy. In February 2017, the DHS issued a memorandum suggesting that parents living in the United States could be prosecuted as smugglers or traffickers of their own children if they attempted to bring their children to the United States—even when their intentions were to protect their children from "conditions in other countries."[58] The next month, then-DHS Secretary Kelly announced he was considering a policy to take children from their parents at the border to deter families from coming to the United States.[59] In the summer of 2017, the Immigration and Customs Enforcement branch of the DHS began targeting for deportation adult family members of unaccompanied children in federal custody who had stepped forward to sponsor children's release, sending waves of fear through immigrant communities.[60] In 2018, as has been well documented, the administration began a process of separating all children and families arriving at the border and to prosecute parents for unlawful entry into the United States. On June 20, 2018, the President issued an Executive Order purporting to end family separation[61] but, as of September 2018, hundreds of the more than 2000 children taken from their parents under the policy remained separated.[62]

Portraying migrant youth as a public safety threat is another prong of the administration's strategy to generate support for its proposed immigration reforms. In particular, the administration has capitalized on individual cases of violence by one gang, MS13, to argue that current immigration policies have allowed the gang to flourish—an argument that flies in the face of DHS's own data.[63] The administration has worked to link these gangs to immigration through particularly dehumanizing language, such as the "infestation" of gang members, who are described as "animals."[63]

Two of the core protections for immigrant youth seeking protection in the United States have also come under attack by the administration. First, the administration has attempted to undo or even end a decades-old, court-ordered agreement,

---

[b] As noted earlier, the program intended to protect "Dreamers"—children brought to the United States at a young age—from deportation and to provide them with authorization to work lawfully was abruptly ended in 2017.

Table 1
Forms of protection from removal

Form of Protection	Description	Where and How Case is Adjudicated	Challenges for Children	Special Concerns
Asylum	Asylum is protection from persecution that is perpetrated on account of a person's race, religion, nationality, political opinion, or membership in a social group	Some cases are heard by asylum officers in a "conference-room"-like setting; others are heard by immigration judges in a formal court proceeding where the child is subject to cross-examination by the government's attorney	Children carry the burden to prove: they have a "well-founded fear of persecution" or experienced past persecution on account of their race, religion, nationality, political opinion, or membership in a social group; and that their persecutor is a government agent or someone the government is unable or unwilling to control. Many of these elements are highly contested and may differ depending on the location where the case is heard	In 2018, the attorney general issued a decision that attempts to limit asylum claims based on domestic violence and gang violence
T nonimmigrant status ("T visa")	Provides 4 y of protection from removal (deportation) for survivors of labor or sex trafficking and provides a path to lawful permanent residence	Adults and children submit a paper-based application; adults must cooperate with law enforcement authorities investigating or prosecuting traffickers	Child victims of labor trafficking often receive less attention from law enforcement and cases of labor trafficking may be underreported and underestimated.[a]	Children granted T status may petition for parents or other family members to receive protection under limited and specific circumstances[b]

(continued on next page)

Table 1
(continued)

Form of Protection	Description	Where and How Case is Adjudicated	Challenges for Children	Special Concerns
U nonimmigrant status ("U visa")	Provides 4 y of protection from removal (deportation) for victims of certain crimes; after 3 y children may apply for lawful permanent residence (LPR) status	Adults and children submit a paper-based application; anyone older than 16 must persuade law enforcement authorities to certify that they cooperated	Only 10,000 "U visas" are granted each year; there is a backlog of approximately 200,000 applications.[c] The backlog results in years-long delays to apply for lawful permanent residence, leaving children in a state of impermanence without access to other benefits that only accrue after 5 y of LPR status	Children granted U status may petition for parents or other family members to receive protection under limited and specific circumstances
Violence Against Women Act (VAWA)	Provides protection for noncitizen children who are abused by a parent or step-parent (similar protection exists for adult abuse survivors)	Applicants submit a paper-based application	Children may apply as the victims of abuse by a parent or step-parent or may receive "derivative" benefits if their parent is granted protection under VAWA	Increasing immigration enforcement efforts in local courts, where victims seek protection against abusers, may result in less protection for abuse survivors
Temporary Protected Status (TPS)	Offers protection for individuals already within the USA who cannot safely return to their country as a result of natural disasters, political upheavals, or other emergency situations.[4]	The federal government invites individuals to apply for TPS status, and requires them to renew status periodically	The protection does not extend to family members living in the home country—for example, the children of TPS recipients, who may remain separated from their parents for years	In December 2016, citizens from 10 different countries were eligible for TPS. The government has since ended TPS for 6 of the 10 countries, and limited TPS for 3 of the[4] remaining countries[d]

Special Immigrant Juvenile Status (SIJS)	SIJS provides protection through age 21 and the ability to pursue LPR status to children who were abused, neglected, or abandoned by a parent, when it is not in their best interests to return to home country	Children appear in state court proceedings—often dependency or custody proceedings—where a state judge must make certain findings as part of the state court case. After receiving those findings, children must apply for SIJS from federal immigration officials	Special immigrant juvenile status ("SIJS") is the only form of protection available solely to children. Yet the process of applying for and receiving SIJS may be the most complex of all forms of protection, requiring proceedings in state court and an application to federal immigration officials	Children from Honduras, El Salvador, Guatemala, and Mexico must wait years until they can apply for LPR status and for authorization to work lawfully in the USA due to backlogs
Deferred Action for Childhood Arrivals (DACA)	Allows children brought to the USA by a certain age, before a certain date, to seek protection from removal for 2-year periods, and to apply for permission to work lawfully	Applicants submit a paper-based application (and significant fees) to immigration authorities	DACA does not provide any path to permanent residency. The hundreds of thousands of children and young adults who applied now fear their applications will be used against them if the program is permanently ended	The ability for DACA holders to renew applications and maintain DACA status, and the ability of other young people to apply for DACA status is the subject of litigation in multiple federal courts, with divergent outcomes. These children and young adults remain in near-intolerable state of uncertainty
Family-based protection	Noncitizen children with a citizen parent, or children of lawful permanent residents or children with more distant relationships to a US citizen, may apply for family-based immigration visas	Paper-based applications	Children of lawful permanent residents or children who have a more distant relationships are subject to numerical caps and may face waits of months or years	The current administration has proposed limiting family-based migration

[a] See Kaufka Walts, Katherine. Child Labor Trafficking in the United States: A Hidden Crime. 2017.
[b] Children's ability to apply for benefits on behalf of family members when applying for T or U status is explained at https://www.uscis.gov/humanitarian/victims-human-trafficking-other-crimes/victims-human-trafficking-t-nonimmigrant-status and https://www.uscis.gov/humanitarian/victims-human-trafficking-other-crimes/victims-human-trafficking-t-nonimmigrant-status respectively.
[c] More information can be found at https://cliniclegal.org/resources/immigration-and-nationality-act-limited-number-u-visas-fiscal-year-2017.
[d] More information about the status of grants of Temporary Protected Status can be found at: https://immigrationforum.org/article/fact-sheet-temporary-protected-status/.

between children's advocates and the government, known as the Flores Settlement agreement. The Flores agreement (and litigation to enforce the agreement over the last 25 years) set forth minimum standards for the care and treatment of immigrant children in government custody, established children's right to be released to parents or family members during their immigration proceedings, and limited the amount of time children can be held in DHS detention facilities.[64] The administration is seeking to upend the Flores agreement so that children who are held with their parents in DHS detention centers and be detained for prolonged or even indefinite periods of time. Second, the administration has attempted to portray a 2008 law known as the William Wilberforce Trafficking Victims Protection Reauthorization Act (TVPRA), passed by a bipartisan Congress and signed by President George W. Bush in 2008, as a "loophole."[65] The 2008 TVPRA provides some of the only protections for unaccompanied children arriving at United States borders, and was intended to help identify possible trafficking victims.

At the same time, the attorney general has made it exponentially more difficult for children to have a fair opportunity to pursue their claims for protection by implementing new case quotas that may make it impossible for immigration judges to fairly consider every case before them[c] and limiting the ability of immigration judges to grant immigrants—including children—time to request and receive immigration benefits from other agencies.[66]

Perhaps most significantly, in 2018 the Attorney General issued a decision that is intended to significantly limit the ability of individuals to win asylum when they are fleeing situations of domestic violence or gang violence.[67] This decision is expected to adversely affect thousands of children and families from Central America, where there is simply no government apparatus to protect survivors of domestic violence, or children at risk of being forcibly recruited into gangs.[67]

Summary: legal considerations

Immigrant children who wish to remain permanently in the United States face a legal process full of risk and uncertainty. It is a process designed primarily for adults, whereby the outcome is not determined by what is in the child's best interests. With so many children seeking protection at our borders, or seeking to avoid removal after a childhood in the United States, the focus should be on establishing procedures and policies that protect them and recognize them first as children. Instead, nearly every protection that exists for immigrant children is under attack.

ADVOCACY

Amid harmful immigration policy and divisive rhetoric, pediatricians are uniquely situated to help inform public debate at local, regional, and national levels regarding the impact of policies on the health and well-being of immigrant children. This section offers strategies and examples for pediatricians to engage in child- and family-centered advocacy from the patient encounter to the public sphere.

Advocacy begins with each child and family at the center. Encounters at the individual level can subsequently inform efforts at broader levels. First and foremost, advocacy must be informed by relevant data. A number of tools exist to evaluate local,

---

[c] Kopan, Tal. Justice Department Rolls out Cas Quotas for Immigration Judges. CNN. April 2, 2018. Available from: https://www.cnn.com/2018/04/02/politics/immigration-judges-quota/index.html. Benner, Katie. Immigration Judges Express Fear that Session's Policy will Impede their Work. NY Times. June 12, 2018. Available from: https://www.nytimes.com/2018/06/12/us/politics/immigration-judges-jeff-sessions.html.

regional, and national demographics with respect to children in immigrant families, including the Kids Count Data Center,[1] the Urban Institute Children of Immigrants Data Tool,[2] and the Migration Policy Institute Migration Data Hub.[3] Second, advocacy can incorporate first-hand clinical experience to humanize the data and connect people to policies. Finally, advocacy should be grounded in evidence-based communication.

When pediatricians engage in advocacy, the intent is to promote the common goal of improved health for all children, including immigrant children. Using evidence-based communication can improve the chance that what is said by the advocate is the message that is received by audiences, whether that audience is the general public or federal policy makers. The Frameworks Institute offers extensive materials, grounded in research, in communications regarding immigration. For instance, using rights-based language in humanitarian arguments can in fact backfire by triggering images of immigrants not abiding by the law. However, emphasizing compassion, dignity, and respect as moral arguments can appeal to shared values.[68] Relying on the science of how messages are received can help to avoid unanticipated reactions and broaden the positive impact of advocacy.

The local level is critical to effect change and support children and families. Within communities, pediatric providers can be an integral part of a network that may facilitate access to critical services. In some communities, efforts to engage in cross-sector collaboration have begun to develop infrastructure. For instance, in North Carolina, Building Integrated Communities (BIC), part of the Latino Migration Project, involves a multiyear community planning process focused on development of relationships between local governments and key stakeholders, including diverse sectors (eg, health, transportation, education, legal, and faith).[69] Each Building Integrated Communities site is able to then develop a tailored approach based on local needs. The BIC initiative is an example of cross-sector collaboration, through which people work to emphasize health by engaging across different fields and the public and private sector to support health and well-being for all.[70]

As many immigration policies are developed and implemented at state and regional levels,[71] advocacy efforts must accordingly include state and regional focus. Coordination within and between regional professional societies can facilitate improved care and access to services for immigrant families. For example, the DC Chapter of the American Academy of Pediatrics developed a robust city-level initiative to coordinate regional advocacy regarding immigrant families.[72] Part of this initiative was to develop a regionally focused immigrant child health toolkit.[73] Regarding legal services, the New York State Immigrant Family Unity Project, funded through the New York State budget, coordinates public defenders to represent immigrants in removal proceedings.[16]

On Capitol Hill, coordinated efforts are critical to effect change. Partnerships between professional organizations and advocacy groups can facilitate shared messaging and enhance the impact (**Table 2**). For instance, after implementation of the Executive Orders in January 2017, rapidly increasing immigration enforcement, the National Immigration Law Center developed a toolkit for health care providers to understand rights and responsibilities to families.[74] Recent efforts to systematically separate families at the southern border were responded to with robust advocacy by organizations across the country using diverse platforms. Pediatricians joined with child welfare experts in other fields to identify the harm of family separation and advocate for policies to prevent family separation in a project led by the Young Center for Immigrant Children's Rights. Ultimately a letter signed by 540 organizations, with representation from all 50 states, DC, and Puerto Rico, was sent to the DHS.[75]

Table 2
Priorities for advocacy: examples from the local level to the public sphere

Local	Regional	National	Public Sphere
• Learn local demographics, learn about local immigrant communities, and invite experts from that community to identify and address local needs • Identify opportunities to facilitate access to high- quality health care for all children even if not eligible for coverage (eg, developing referral networks with free and low-cost clinics, hospital sponsorship for children with medical complexity) • Advocate for local policy that prioritizes access to affordable housing and green spaces • Develop strategies to enhance access to free or low-cost legal services • Collaborate with local legal services organizations to develop a "know your rights" pamphlet that addresses the issues we have included in this article, and make it available to all clients in various languages • Protect the rights of immigrant children to free public K-12 education and coordinate with public schools to meet educational needs and build resources • Partner across sectors to build coalitions (eg, medical-legal)	• Prioritize health coverage for all children regardless of immigration status at the state level, as exists in several states • Engage with state professional societies to coordinate advocacy efforts • Work with state legislators to ensure fair state immigration policies	• Prioritize the right to protection for children and families seeking safe haven, including avoiding separation of parents from children for any period of time, avoiding detention of children, and ensuring child welfare throughout the immigration process • Prioritize eligibility for health coverage regardless of immigration status • Support legislation that provides legal representation to children in immigration proceedings • Advocate for an explicit "best interests of the child" mandate • Engage with national professional societies (eg, AAP, AAFP) to increase the reach of efforts	• Rely on evidence-based communication strategies • Engage in multiple spheres, including print media and social media • Coordinate with allied organizations and sectors to garner greater impact • Avoid stereotypes when communicating about immigrant families • Embrace storytelling to demonstrate need for policy change (protecting all confidential/personal information)

Although policy remains in flux, pediatric providers are a credible and critical part of advocacy for federal policy that supports the health and well-being of immigrant children and families.

In a changing world, advocacy efforts continue to expand within the public sphere. In the earned media (eg, editorials and opinion pieces, interviews, and live appearances), pediatric providers can contribute evidence-based material that adds cross-sector credibility and strength to these efforts. Social media (eg, Facebook and Twitter) offers additional opportunities to reach the public with credible messages. Some pediatricians have incorporated additional media-based strategies to connect with and support special populations (eg, "Las Doctoras Recomiendan," a Podcast created by pediatricians and supported by a grant from the American Academy of Pediatrics to share evidence-based health information with Latino families[76]). A broad spectrum of advocacy efforts can ultimately engage diverse audiences to support the health and well-being of all children and families.

SUMMARY

Advocacy regarding children in immigrant families is inspired by compassion, informed by data, and advanced through determination and cross-sector collaboration. As the population of children in immigrant families evolves and relevant immigration and health policies emerge, health care providers have an essential responsibility to engage in advocacy efforts at individual, local, regional, national, and transnational levels. Ultimately, when all children can achieve their optimal health and well-being, our communities collectively benefit.

REFERENCES

1. Annie E Casey Foundation. Kids count data center 2018. Available at: http://datacenter.kidscount.org/. Accessed June 11, 2018.
2. Bivand Erdal M, Oeppen C. Forced to leave? The discursive and analytical significance of describing migration as forced and voluntary. J Ethn Migr Stud 2018;44(6):981–98.
3. Gheasi M, Nijkamp P. A brief overview of international migration motives and impacts, with specific reference to FDI. Economies 2017;5(31). https://doi.org/10.3390/economies5030031.
4. Hipsamn F, Meissner D. Immigration in the United States: new economic, social, political landscapes with legislative reform on the horizon. Washington, DC: Migration Information Source; 2013. Available at: https://www.migrationpolicy.org/article/immigration-united-states-new-economic-social-political-landscapes-legislative-reform. Accessed June 11, 2018.
5. FitzGerald DS, Cook-Martin D. The geopolitical origins of the U.S. immigration act of 1965. Migration Information Source Web site 2015. Available at: https://www.migrationpolicy.org/article/geopolitical-origins-us-immigration-act-1965. Accessed June 11, 2018.
6. Pierce S, Bolter J, Selee A. Trump's first year on immigration policy: rhetoric vs. reality. Washington, DC: Migration Policy Institute; 2018. Available at: https://www.migrationpolicy.org/research/trump-first-year-immigration-policy-rhetoric-vs-reality. Accessed March 16, 2019.
7. Potochnick S, Chen JH, Perrera K. Local-level immigration enforcement and food insecurity risk among Hispanic immigrant families with children: national-level evidence. J Immigr Minor Health 2017;19(5):1042–9.

8. Novak N, Geronimus A, Martinez Cardoso A. Change in birth outcomes among infants born to Latina mothers after a major immigration raid. Int J Epidemiol 2017;46(3). https://doi.org/10.1093/ije/dyw346.

9. Lopez WD, Kruger DJ, Delva J, et al. Health implications of an immigration raid: Findings from a Latino community in the midwestern United States. J Immigr Minor Health 2017;19(3):702–8.

10. Hatzenbuehler M, Prin S, Flake M, et al. Immigration policies and mental health morbidity among Latinos: a state-level analysis. Soc Sci Med 2017;174:169–78.

11. Artiga S, Ubri P. Living in an immigrant family in America: how fear and toxic stress are affecting daily life, well-being, and health. Washginton, DC: Henry J. Kaiser Foundation. Available at: https://www.kff.org/disparities-policy/issue-brief/living-in-an-immigrant-family-in-america-how-fear-and-toxic-stress-are-affecting-daily-life-well-being-health/. Accessed March 16, 2019.

12. Garner AS, Shonkoff JP. Early childhood adversity, toxic stress, and the role of the pediatrician: translating developmental science into lifelong health. Pediatrics 2012;129:e224.

13. Centers for Disease Control and Prevention. Social determinants of health 2018. Available at: https://www.cdc.gov/socialdeterminants/. Accessed August 21, 2018.

14. Centers for Disease Control and Prevention. Health equity | resources | tools and resources | National Center for Chronic Disease Prevention and Health Promotion | CDC. Health Equity Web site. 2018. Available at: https://www.cdc.gov/chronicdisease/healthequity/index.htm. Accessed September 7, 2018.

15. Health coverage of immigrants. 2018. The Henry J. Kaiser Family Foundation Web site. Available at: https://www.kff.org/disparities-policy/fact-sheet/health-coverage-of-immigrants/. Accessed March 16, 2019.

16. Health care coverage maps. National Immigration Law Center Web site. 2018. Available at: https://www.nilc.org/issues/health-care/healthcoveragemaps/. Accessed September 7, 2018.

17. Avila R. Language and immigrant status effects on disparities in Hispanic children's health status and access to health care. Matern Child Health J 2013; 17(3):423, 423.

18. Burgos AE, Schetzina KE, Dixon LB, et al. Importance of generational status in examining access to and utilization of health care services by Mexican American children. Pediatrics 2005;115(3):e322. Available at: http://pediatrics.aappublications.org/content/115/3/e322.abstract.

19. Chilton L, Handal G, Paz-Soldan G, et al. Providing care for immigrant, migrant, and border children. Pediatrics 2013;131:E2034. Available at: https://pediatrics.aappublications.org/content/131/6/e2028. Accessed July 6, 2018.

20. Reza M, Amin MS, Sgro A, et al. Oral health status of immigrant and refugee children in North America: a scoping review. J Can Dent Assoc 2016;82:g3. Available at: http://www.jcda.ca/g3. Accessed July 6, 2018.

21. Gupta RP, de Wit ML, McKeown D. The impact of poverty on the current and future health status of children. Paediatr Child Health 2007;12(8):667–72. Available at: https://www.ncbi.nlm.nih.gov/pubmed/19030444.

22. Semega J, Fontenot K, Kollar M. Income and poverty in the United States: 2016. U.S. Census Bureau; 2017. p. 60–259. Current Population Reports.

23. Thomas KJ. Familial influences on poverty among young children in black immigrant, U.S.-born black, and nonblack immigrant families. Demography 2011; 48(2):437–60.

24. Coleman-Jensen A, Rabbitt MP, Gregory CA, et al. Household food security in the United States in 2016. United States Department of Agriculture, Economic Research Service; 2017. https://www.ers.usda.gov/webdocs/publications/84973/err-237.pdf?v=42979. Accessed March 15, 2019.

25. Council on Community Pediatrics, Committee on Nutrition. Promoting food security for all children. Pediatrics 2015;136(5):1431.

26. Chilton M, Black MM, Berkowitz C, et al. Food insecurity and risk of poor health among US-born children of immigrants. American Journal of Public Health 2009; 99(3):556–62.

27. Johnson-Motoyama M. Does a paradox exist in child well-being risks among foreign-born Latinos, U.S.-born Latinos, and whites? Findings from 50 California cities. Child Abuse Negl 2014;38(6):1061–72.

28. Kalil A, Chen J. Mothers' citizenship status and household food insecurity among low-income children of immigrants. New Directions For Child And Adolescent Development 2008;2008(121):43–62.

29. Ortega AN, Horwitz SM, Fang H, et al. Documentation status and parental concerns about development in young US children of Mexican origin. Academic Pediatrics 2009;9(4):278–82.

30. Batalova J, Fix M, Greenberg M. Chilling effects: The expected public charge rule and its impact on legal immigrant families' public benefits use. Available at: https://www.migrationpolicy.org/research/chilling-effects-expected-public-charge-rule-impact-legal-immigrant-families. Updated 2018. Accessed March 15, 2019.

31. Olivas MA. Plyler v Doe: Still guaranteeing unauthorized immigrant children's right to attend U.S. public schools. Migration Information Source Web site. 2010. Available at: https://www.migrationpolicy.org/article/plyler-v-doe-still-guaranteeing-unauthorized-immigrant-childrens-right-attend-us-public. Accessed September 12, 2018.

32. Plyler v Doe, No. 80-1538. 457 U.S. 202. Argued December 1, 1981. Decided June 15, 1982.

33. US Department of Education. Schools' civil rights obligations to English learner students and limited English proficient parents 2018. Available at: https://www2.ed.gov/about/offices/list/ocr/ellresources.html. Accessed July 18, 2018.

34. American Immigration Council. Public education for immigrant students: understanding Plyler v. Doe. 2016. Available at: https://www.americanimmigrationcouncil.org/research/plyler-v-doe-public-education-immigrant-students. Accessed July 18, 2018.

35. Danso K. Nativity and health disparities: predictors of immigrant health. Soc Work Public Health 2016;31(3):175–87.

36. Hummer RA, Hernandez EM. The effect of educational attainment on adult mortality in the United States. Popul Bull 2013;68(1):1. Available at: https://www.ncbi.nlm.nih.gov/pubmed/25995521.

37. Taylor RJ, Forsythe-Brown I, Mouzon DM, et al. Prevalence and correlates of everyday discrimination among black Caribbeans in the United States: the impact of nativity and country of origin. Ethn Health 2017;1–21. https://doi.org/10.1080/13557858.2017.1346785. Available at: https://www-tandfonline-com.proxygw.wrlc.org/doi/full/10.1080/13557858.2017.1346785. Accessed July 18, 2018.

38. Pérez DJ, Fortuna L, Alegria M. Prevalence and correlates of everyday discrimination among U.S. Latinos. J Community Psychol 2008;36(4):421–33. Available at: https://onlinelibrary.wiley.com/doi/abs/10.1002/jcop.20221. Accessed September 7, 2018.

39. Carlisle S, Stone A. Effects of perceived discrimination and length of residency on the health of foreign-born populations. J Racial Ethn Health Disparities 2015;2(4): 434–44. Available at: https://www.ncbi.nlm.nih.gov/pubmed/26863551.

40. Chan WY, Latzman RD. Racial discrimination, multiple group identities, and civic beliefs among immigrant adolescents. Cultur Divers Ethnic Minor Psychol 2015; 21(4):527–32. Available at: https://psycnet.apa.org/record/2014-56036-001. Accessed September 7, 2018.

41. Flores E, Tschann JM, Dimas JM, et al. Perceived racial/ethnic discrimination, posttraumatic stress symptoms, and health risk behaviors among Mexican American adolescents. J Couns Psychol 2010;57(3):264–73. Available at: https:// psycnet.apa.org/record/2010-14017-002. Accessed July 18, 2018.

42. Tummala-Narra P, Claudius M. Perceived discrimination and depressive symptoms among immigrant-origin adolescents. Cultur Divers Ethnic Minor Psychol 2013;19(3):257–69.

43. Yoo HC, Castro KS. Does nativity status matter in the relationship between perceived racism and academic performance of Asian American college students? J Coll Stud Dev 2011;52(2):234–45. Available at: https://muse.jhu.edu/ article/431418. Accessed July 18, 2018.

44. Bashir SA. Home is where the harm is: inadequate housing as a public health crisis. Am J Public Health 2002;92(5):733–8. Available at: http://ajph. aphapublications.org/cgi/content/abstract/92/5/733.

45. Rauh VA, Landrigan PJ, Claudio L. Housing and health: intersection of poverty and environmental exposures. Ann N Y Acad Sci 2008;1136:276–88. Available at: http://europepmc.org/abstract/med/18579887. Accessed August 4, 2018.

46. Maxwell AE, Young S, Crespi CM, et al. Social determinants of health in the Mixtec and Zapotec community in Ventura county, California. Int J Equity Health 2015;14. https://doi.org/10.1186/s12939-015-0148-0.

47. Arcury TA, Trejo G, Suerken CK, et al. Stability of household and housing characteristics among farmworker families in North Carolina: implications for health. J Immigr Minor Health 2017;19(2):398–406. Accessed August 4, 2018.

48. Cox DTC, Shanahan DF, Hudson HL, et al. Doses of neighborhood nature: The benefits for mental health of living with nature. BioScience 2017;67(2):147–55. Available at: https://academic.oup.com/bioscience/article/67/2/147/2900179. Accessed August 4, 2018.

49. Keniger LE, Gaston KJ, Irvine KN, et al. What are the benefits of interacting with nature? Int J Environ Res Public Health 2013;10(3):913–35. Available at: https:// www.ncbi.nlm.nih.gov/pmc/articles/PMC3709294/. Accessed August 4, 2018.

50. Hordyk SR, Hanley J, Richard E. "Nature is there; it's free": urban greenspace and the social determinants of health of immigrant families. Health Place 2015;34: 74–82.

51. U.S. Department of Housing and Urban Development. Fair housing laws and presidential executive orders. Available at: https://www.hud.gov/program_ offices/fair_housing_equal_opp/fair_housing_and_related_law. Accessed March 16, 2019.

52. U.S. Code Title 8. ALIENS AND NATIONALITY Chapter 12. IMMIGRATION AND NATIONALITY Subchapter II. IMMIGRATION Part IV. Inspection, Apprehension, Examination, Exclusion, and Removal Section 1232. Enhancing efforts to combat the trafficking of children.

53. U.S. Code Title 8. ALIENS AND NATIONALITY Chapter 12. IMMIGRATION AND NATIONALITY Subchapter II. IMMIGRATION Part IV. Inspection, Apprehension,

Examination, Exclusion, and Removal Section 1232. Enhancing efforts to combat the trafficking of children.

54. GAO. Unaccompanied Children: HHS Should Improve Monitoring and Information Sharing Policies to Enhance Child Advocate Program Effectiveness. 2016 (Report found that over 70% of Child Advocate recommendations are accepted by agencies making decisions about children). Available at: https://www.gao.gov/products/GAO-16-367. Accessed March 16, 2019.

55. U.S. Code Title 8. ALIENS AND NATIONALITY Chapter 12. IMMIGRATION AND NATIONALITY Subchapter II. IMMIGRATION Part IX. Miscellaneous Section 1362. Right to counsel.

56. In re Gault, No. 116. 387 U.S. 1. Argued December 6, 1966. Decided May 15, 1967.

57. For more information see Available at: https://www.aclu.org/blog/immigrants-rights/deportation-and-due-process/immigrant-children-do-not-have-right-attorney. Accessed March 16, 2019. C.J.L.G. v. Sessions. 880 F.3d 1122. (9th Cir. 2018).

58. DHS Secretary Kelly. DHS memorandum: implementing the President's border security and immigration enforcement improvement policies. Washington, DC: US Department of Homeland Security; 2017.

59. Gajanan M. Homeland security chief says he's considering separating immigrant children from parents 2017. Available at: http://time.com/4692899/homeland-security-john-kelly-separate-children-parents-immigration/. Accessed March 16, 2019.

60. Burke G. Feds will now target relatives. AP news 2017. Available at: https://apnews.com/291d565801984005886f5a22c800fee6/Feds-will-now-target-relatives-who-smuggled-in-children. Accessed March 16, 2019.

61. Valverde M. Donald Trump's Executive Order ending his administration's separation of immigrant families. Politifact 2018. Available at: https://www.politifact.com/truth-o-meter/article/2018/jun/25/donald-trumps-executive-order-ending-his-administr/. Accessed March 16, 2019.

62. Shapiro L, Manas S. How many migrant children are still separated from their families. Washington Post 2018. Available at: https://www.washingtonpost.com/graphics/2018/local/tracking-migrant-family-separation/?utm_term=.c391ae8c5883.

63. Sahil C, Ma J, Thompson SA. MS-13 is far from the "infestation" Trump describes. NY Times 2018. Available at: https://www.nytimes.com/interactive/2018/06/27/opinion/trump-ms13-immigration.html.

64. Flynn M. Federal judge denies Trump administration's request to indefinitely detain families. Washington Post 2018. Available at: https://www.washingtonpost.com/news/morning-mix/wp/2018/07/10/federal-judge-denies-trump-administrations-request-to-indefinitely-detain-families/?utm_term=.fb5c806ea08a.

65. Mark M. The Trump administration keeps blaming "loopholes" in immigration law for its family separation policy. Business Insider 2018. Available at: https://www.businessinsider.com/immigration-loopholes-asylum-law-trump-administration-congress-2018-6.

66. U.S. Department of Justice Office of the Attorney General. 27 I&N Dec. 271 (A.G. 2018). Matter of CASTRO-TUM, Respondent. Decided by Attorney General May 17, 2018.

67. Matter of A-B-. 27 I&N Dec. 316 (2018) (holding that "generally, claims by aliens pertaining to domestic violence or gang violence perpetrated by

nongovernmental actors will not qualify for asylum"). Available at: https://www.justice.gov/eoir/page/file/1070866/download. Accessed March 16, 2019.

68. O'Neil M, Kendall-Taylor N, Bales SN. Finish the story on immigration: a Frame-Works MessageMemo. Washington, DC: FrameWorks Institute; 2014.

69. UNC Global. The Latino Migration Project. Building Integrated Communities. 2018. Available at: https://migration.unc.edu/programs/bic/. Accessed June 29, 2018.

70. Robert Wood Johnson Foundation. Fostering cross-sector collaboration to improve well-being. 2018. Available at: https://www.rwjf.org/en/cultureofhealth/taking-action/fostering-cross-sector-collaboration.html. Accessed June 29, 2018.

71. Philbin MM, Flake M, Hatzenbuehler ML, et al. State-level immigration and immigrant-focused policies as drivers of L health disparities in the United States. Soc Sci Med 2018;199:29–38.

72. DC Chapter of the American Academy of Pediatrics. DC Chapter initiatives: immigrant health. 2018. Available at: http://aapdc.org/chapter-initiatives/immigrant-health/. Accessed July 1, 2018.

73. Immigrant Child Health Committee of the DC Chapter of the American Academy of Pediatrics. DC Chapter immigrant child health toolkit. 2018. Available at: http://aapdc.org/toolkit/immigranthealth/. Accessed July 1, 2018.

74. National Immigration Law Center. Health care provider and immigration enforcement: Know your rights, know your patients' rights. 2017. Available at: https://www.nilc.org/issues/immigration-enforcement/healthcare-provider-and-patients-rights-imm-enf/. Accessed July 1, 2018.

75. Renewed appeal from experts in child welfare, juvenile justice and child development to halt the separation of children from parents at the border. 2018. Available at: https://static1.squarespace.com/static/597ab5f3bebafb0a625aaf45/t/5b196fbf70a6ade9adfb3377/1528393664012/REV_2018_06_07_Child+Welfare+Juvenile+Justice+Opposition+to+Parent+Child+Separation+%281%29.pdf. Accessed July 1, 2018.

76. Las Doctoras Recomiendan. Las doctoras recomiendan. 2018.

Acculturative Stress and Mental Health

Implications for Immigrant-Origin Youth

Selcuk R. Sirin, PhD[a],*, Esther Sin, MA[b], Clare Clingain, BS[c],
Lauren Rogers-Sirin, PhD[d]

KEYWORDS

- Immigrants • Mental health • Acculturation • Adolescents
- Psychological development • Social development

KEY POINTS

- Growing antiimmigrant sentiment in the United States create many developmental challenges for immigrant origin youth.
- Immigrant youth experience high levels of acculturative stress, which have been linked to their negative mental health trajectories.
- Multiple psychological and environmental factors may serve as protective factors against the negative effects of acculturative stress on mental health outcomes.
- The authors provide evidence from their longitudinal study that empirically demonstrates implications of acculturative stress on key mental health outcomes during adolescence.

Today more than 1 in 4 children in the United States are children and youth in immigrant families, and this figure is expected to reach 1 in 3 by midcentury.[1] Despite their increasing numbers, until very recently we lack empirically validated understanding of mental health for this important section of the society. In an effort to address this gap in the literature, the authors rely on a new conceptual framework to provide a brief overview of the current immigration debate, as it affects immigrant origin youth.

Disclosure Statement: The authors do not have any affiliation with any commercial companies that may have an interest in this subject.
[a] Department of Applied Psychology, Steinhardt School of Culture, Education, and Human Development, New York University, 246 Greene Street, Room 404, New York, NY 10003, USA;
[b] Department of Applied Psychology, Steinhardt School of Culture, Education, and Human Development, New York University, 246 Greene Street, Room 621E, New York, NY 10003, USA;
[c] Department of Applied Statistics, Social Science, and Humanities, Steinhardt School of Culture, Education, and Human Development, New York University, 246 Greene Street, Room 621E, New York, NY 10003, USA; [d] Department of Psychology, College of Staten Island, The City University of New York, 2800 Victory Boulevard, 4S Room 233, Staten Island, NY 10314, USA
* Corresponding author.
E-mail address: sirins@nyu.edu

Next, they present results from their longitudinal studies to provide empirical evidence of the negative influence acculturative stress can have on mental health outcomes. Finally, they discuss the clinical implications of their work with an emphasis on meeting the mental health needs of youth in immigrant families.

One of the rare theoretic models specifically designed to understand immigrant youth development is the integrative risk and resilience model (**Fig. 1**). This conceptual framework, originally developed by García-Coll and colleagues,[2] highlights the positive adaptation of youth in immigrant families (eg, developmental tasks, psychological adjustment, and acculturative tasks) and the global- and developmental-level contexts that shape youth experiences. Youth in immigrant families face several contextual challenges to successful adaptation[3] and as shown in **Fig. 1**, influences from 4 levels, including global, sociopolitical, microsystem, and individual influences that contribute independently, or in interaction with each other, to shape the group and individual variation in adaptation.

Youth in immigrant families experience the typical developmental challenges of growing up that their nonimmigrant peers do, but they also have to negotiate multiple cultural demands from their home and host cultures. This process of acculturation at both the micro- and the macro-levels has implications for their social, emotional, and psychological development.[4] At the micro-level, youth in immigrant families have to adjust to a new language, a new education system, and may have to act as language brokers for their parents, or work after school to financially support their family.[4,5] At the macro-level, they are more likely to live in poverty, to face uncomfortable scrutiny due to their legal status in the country, and face the threat of family separation and deportation.[6] Combined, these micro and macro factors have the potential to negatively affect the mental health of youth in immigrant families.

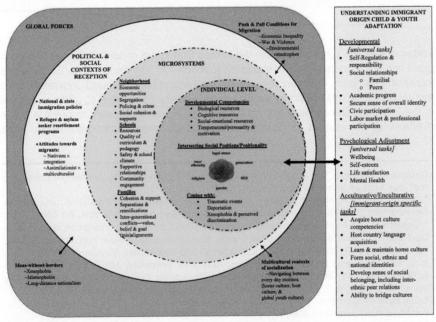

Fig. 1. Integrative risk and resilience model for the adaptation of youth in immigrant families. (*From* Suárez-Orozco C, Motti-Stefanidi F, Marks A, et al. An integrative risk and resilience model for understanding the adaptation of immigrant-origin children and youth. Am Psychol 2018;73(6):781–96.)

GROWING ANTIIMMIGRANT RHETORIC

Outside of the family and school environments, youth in immigrant families face anti-immigrant sentiment and are at risk of discrimination as a result of their immigrant and cultural identities.[7] Institutional and cultural barriers often prevent immigrants from fully participating as citizens, creating a social stigma of being "foreign" and "other" compared with mainstream American culture. Immigration has always been a divisive topic, but with the 2016 general election it has become as central and heated as the debate over the economy. Trump's election has turned extreme rhetoric about immigration and immigrants into public policy, affecting millions of youth in immigrant families. A recent review by the Migration Policy Institute[8] shows that there are 4 areas where the Trump administration has made life for youth in immigrant families more difficult (**Box 1**).

The implications of these policy changes are 2-fold. On the one hand, there is evidence that, despite political rhetoric, most of the US public continues to have sympathy for immigrants overall.[9] There is also growing public backlash toward some of the most controversial policies, such as family separation. According to a survey by Quinnipiac University, two-thirds of Americans oppose a policy that has led to more than 2000 children being separated from their parents at the US border.[10] Despite these bright spots, the growing antiimmigrant political rhetoric has the risk of normalizing discrimination and violence toward a vulnerable population, which in turn increases their acculturative stress.[9] In the next section, the authors consider how such stress affects youth in immigrant families and their mental health outcomes.

MENTAL HEALTH IMPLICATIONS OF ACCULTURATION STRESS

Acculturation is a complicated and dynamic process of changes on multiple levels including individual, family, and cultural.[11] It is considered one of the key developmental processes for youth in immigrant families, and it can be broadly defined as the changes that occur in an individual or group of individuals as a result of contact with different cultures and social systems.[12,13] Two dominant models have been proposed to explain the acculturation process: unidimensional model and bidimensional model. Earlier studies have conceptualized the process of acculturation as a

---

Box 1
What has changed for immigrants during Trump's presidency?

1. Enhanced immigrant enforcement that resulted in separation of children from families and expanding deportation raids throughout the country.

2. Cut back on humanitarian programs that resulted in the lowest number of refugees admitted to the United States over the past 30 years and termination of Temporary Protection Status for more than 300,000 individuals who seek refuge in the United States due to conflict in their home countries.

3. Increased vetting and obstacles for legal immigration that aims to significantly decrease the number of individuals who can get visas to legally enter and work in the country, as well as move through the citizenship path.

4. Worked to end Deferred Action for Childhood Arrivals, a program currently providing protection for more than 700,000 unauthorized children.

Data from Migration Policy Institute. U.S. Immigration policy under trump: deep changes and lasting impacts. 2018. Available at: https://www.migrationpolicy.org/research/us-immigration-policy-trump-deep-changes-impacts. Accessed October 1, 2018.

unidimensional model, also known as the assimilation model, which assumes that as an individual/group acculturates to the host culture, they would let go of the heritage culture's beliefs, values, and attitudes.[14] The underlying assumption of the unidimensional model is that the individual/group changes in a linear relation from the home culture to the host culture, and the strengthening of one culture requires a weakening of the other. In contrast to the unidimensional model, a bidimensional model places the maintenance of the home culture and the adoption of the host culture independent of one another.[15–18] The underlying assumption of the bidimensional model is that individual/groups can adopt the practices of the host culture without giving up the practices of the home culture. Most scholars now agree that acculturation should not be conceptualized as a unidirectional process but as a bidimensional process.[11]

Depending on how one acculturates,[11] there may be a negative relation between acculturation strategy and mental health (**Box 2**). Support for this relation seems to depend highly on whether the researchers used a unidimensional or bidimensional model. When one examines unidimensional acculturation, greater adherence to the host culture's values predicts positive mental health outcomes.[19] Within the bidimensional framework, however, youth in immigrant families who either identify positively with both host culture and culture of origin (integrated) or identify only with culture of origin (separated) tend to have better mental health outcomes than those who do not identify with either culture (marginalized).[20] Integrated youth report fewer anxious-depressive and somatic symptoms than their counterparts.[21,22] Among immigrants who are diagnosed with major depressive disorder, those who are integrated have fewer symptoms than those who are separated, who in turn have fewer symptoms than their assimilated counterparts.[23] Thus, understanding the acculturation process in the lives of immigrant youth is critical in understanding their overall psychological health.

Acculturation is a challenging and stressful process, and various studies have demonstrated the negative impact of acculturative stressors on the mental health of this population.[21] The unique stressors that immigrants experience is referred to as acculturative stress. A variety of factors may contribute to acculturative stress, such

---

Box 2
Mental health outcomes by acculturation strategy

Assimilation

- More depressive symptoms than separated for those clinically diagnosed with major depressive disorder[23]

Integration

- Fewer anxious-depressive symptoms than all counterparts[21,22]
- Fewer somatic symptoms than all counterparts[21,22]
- Better mental health outcomes than marginalized[20]
- Fewer depressive symptoms than separated and assimilated for those clinically diagnosed with major depressive disorder[23]

Separation

- Fewer depressive symptoms than assimilated for those clinically diagnosed with major depressive disorder[23]

Marginalization

- Tend to have worst mental health outcome[20]

as separation from families, reasons for immigrating, and documentation status.[24] Youth in immigrant families may also experience additional stress due to the fact that many often act as cultural negotiators between family and teacher expectations. Teachers sometimes view immigrant students as less competent and immigrant parents as being indifferent and unsupportive to their children's education. Youth in immigrant families often find themselves trying to facilitate conversations between their teachers and parents despite the language and cultural difference.[25]

High levels of acculturative stress have been linked to negative mental health trajectories among youth in immigrant families.[26] For example, in a sample of Korean immigrant youth, greater acculturative stress is linked to higher depression and lower self-esteem.[27] Yet some researchers suggest that one must examine acculturation and acculturative stress simultaneously to understand how it affects mental health. Although not identifying with the mainstream culture is linked to greater depressive symptoms for Asian Americans, this relation disappears once acculturative stress is accounted for.[28] Thus, acculturative stress may serve as a risk factor. The next section discusses the protective factors that buffer the negative effects of acculturative stress on mental health outcomes.

PROTECTIVE FACTORS

Multiple psychological and environmental factors may serve as protective factors against the negative effects of acculturative stress on mental health outcomes (**Fig. 2**). Such factors can serve to mitigate or exacerbate the role of acculturative stress on mental health symptoms. For example, having a strong ethnic identity—the degree to which one identifies with one's ethnic group—can lower the risk of developing a lifetime psychological disorder among youth in immigrant families.[29] Similarly, social support from host culture friends may nullify the negative association of the marginalization acculturation strategy and the psychological adaptation of youth.[30] That is, youth who report higher levels of support from friends may not exhibit any psychological maladaptation associated with marginalized acculturation. At moderate levels of support, youth may still experience poor psychological adaptation, but at a smaller magnitude than those with little support.[30] Therefore, the contexts in

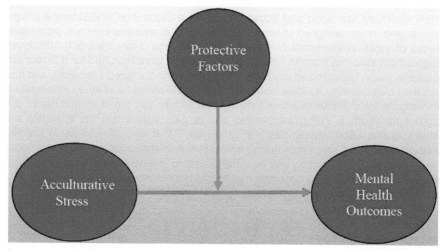

Fig. 2. Protective factors of mental health. Protective Factors: Ethnic identity[29]; Social support;[30,31] Coping skills;[32,33] Self-esteem;[34] Family cohesion.[35]

which youth garner local friendships—schools and neighborhoods—are crucial not only for their social development but also for their psychological development.

Some studies have found the positive role of social support in buffering the relation between acculturative stress and mental health outcomes. Specifically, higher levels of social support protect immigrant youth from experiencing psychological symptoms associated with acculturative stress.[31] Youth who receive high levels of social support report fewer psychological symptoms compared with those with low levels of social support.

Stronger psychological coping skills and higher self-esteem may also buffer against the negative association between acculturative stress and psychological well-being.[32] That is, immigrants who can better manage their stresses in general may not be as psychologically affected by acculturative stress. In addition to coping, one's identification with the home culture may further moderate the relation between acculturative stress and psychological distress. Immigrants who strongly identify with their ethnic heritage tend not to use forbearance coping (ie, hiding one's problems). Youth in immigrant families who use forbearance coping show a weaker association between acculturative stress and psychological distress.[33] In addition to coping skills, higher self-esteem may protect them from acculturative stress-related mental health symptoms.[34] Regardless of one's socioeconomic status or age of immigration, youth who have a better view of themselves tend to have greater psychological well-being than those with poor self-esteem.

Finally, family cohesion can protect youth in immigrant families from depressive symptoms associated with acculturative stress, such that youth who report greater family cohesion experience fewer depressive symptoms than youth who experience greater family conflict.[35] Overall, varying forms of social support, whether from family or friends, should be considered as crucial parts to immigrant youths' well-being and adaptation to a new environment. With shifts in the global forces via increased family separation and ostracization of immigrants in the era of Trump, many of these protective factors in the microsystems that are nested in the larger global context are threatened, which, at the individual level, puts immigrant youth at risk for poorer psychological outcomes.[3]

FINDINGS FROM THE NEW YORK CITY ACADEMIC AND SOCIAL ENGAGEMENT STUDY

New York City Academic and Social Engagement Study (NYCASES) was a 3-wave longitudinal study designed to understand the educational and psychological trajectories of youth in immigrant families in urban settings. More than 500 10th grade high school students from 14 New York City schools were recruited for a 3-year longitudinal study. Using mixed methods of surveys, semistructured interviews, and map drawing methodology for data collection, NYCASES offered a unique opportunity to investigate the complex relations between the factors that affect mental health outcomes for youth in immigrant families and to gain insight into the strengths and stressors that affect mental health in urban life.[36,37] It also allowed us to examine key developmental processes during adolescence, in particular acculturation, acculturative stress, and identity, and how they relate to mental health outcomes. Below the authors provide a brief description of the study methods (**Box 3, Table 1**) and overall findings from the study as it relates to their mental health.

RESULTS
Mental Health Outcomes

A major finding of NYCASES was that internalizing mental health symptoms declined significantly over time during the high school years. Both linear and quadratic slopes were explored as predictors of growth in the outcome variables to determine the growth pattern that best represented change over time. Overall, 3 types of mental health symptoms—withdrawn/depressed, anxious/depressed, and somatic symptoms—decreased over time between 10th and 12th grade, although in different patterns.[42–44] The linear model fit best for withdrawn/depressed symptoms, meaning, withdrawn/depressed symptoms decreased between each time of measurement, $\beta = -0.06$, $P<.001$. On the other hand, a quadratic model fit best for anxious/depressed ($\beta = 0.06$, $P<.01$) and somatic symptoms ($\beta = 0.06$, $P<.01$), with both following a curved pattern in which symptoms decreased, plateaued, and then began to increase again by the 12th grade. All together, these findings show that mental health among immigrant high school students improves overtime, but with variation. Given our multigenerational, multiethnic group sample, these results provide insight into the role of acculturative stress in the expression of psychological symptoms over time.

Trajectories of Mental Health Symptoms

Despite an overall decline in mental health symptoms during adolescence, it is also found that acculturative stress independently increased risk for mental health symptoms over time.[37] Specifically, during the high school years, as acculturative stress increased, withdrawn/depressed ($\beta = 0.05$, $P<.001$), somatic ($\beta = 0.07$, $P<.001$), and anxious/depressed symptoms ($\beta = 0.10$, $P<.001$) also increased significantly. These findings confirm the deleterious role acculturative stress can play in development and mental health among immigrant populations.[42–44] These results also affirm the need for culturally competent professionals to work with immigrant youth.

The results also demonstrated that social support networks can buffer the negative effect of acculturative stress on mental health. Youth with high levels of support tended to have fewer anxious/depressive ($\beta = -0.07$, $P<.01$) and withdrawn symptoms ($\beta = -0.15$, $P<.001$).[26] Moreover, for youth with lower levels of support, the relation between acculturative stress and anxious/depressive symptoms was stronger

---

Box 3
Measures from New York City Academic and Social Engagement Study

Acculturative Stress: Societal, Attitudinal, Familial, and Environmental (SAFE)—Revised Short Form[38]
- "It bothers me that family members I am close to do not understand my new American values"
- 0 (not at all stressful) to 4 (very stressful)

Mental Health: Youth Self-Report[39]
- Withdrawn symptoms: "I keep from getting involved with others"
- Anxious-depressive symptoms: "I feel that no one loves me"
- Somatic symptoms: "I feel overtired without reason"
- 0 (never) to 2 (very often)

Social Support: Adapted from interview protocol for Longitudinal Immigrant Student Adaptation Study[40]
- "Are there people you can talk to about your feelings"
- 0 (definitely not) to 4 (definitely yes)

Ethnic identification: Collective Self-esteem Scale–Race[41]
- Private collective self-esteem: "In general, I am glad to be a member of my racial/ethnic group"
- Importance to identity: "In general, belonging to my racial/ethnic group is an important part of my self-image"

Table 1 Sample information for New York City Academic and Social Engagement Study			
	Female	Male	Total
Gender	56% (n = 186)	44% (n = 146)	332
	First Generation	Second Generation	Total
Generation Status	48% (n = 159)	52% (n = 173)	332

(Z = 8.11, P<.01) than for youth with higher levels of support (Z = 4.68, P<.01). Thus, social support provides a buffering effect for anxious/depressive symptoms, but not withdrawn symptoms.

The protective nature of social support may be of particular importance to first-generation youth who, on average, experience higher levels of acculturative stress (F(1,265) = 39.15, P<.001) and withdrawn symptoms (F(1,266) = 4.36, P<.05) compared with second-generation youth (see also **Fig. 2**).[37] Our findings run contrary to the "immigrant paradox" literature, which suggests that second-generation youth exhibit poorer mental health outcomes than first-generation.[20]

The stressors for first-generation immigrants, which center on learning a new language, family separation and disruption, and adjusting to a new culture, may have greater implications for mental health as opposed to the challenges experienced by second-generation immigrants.

Racial and Ethnic Group Differences

In their study, the authors also investigated whether there are important distinctions between Asian and Latino immigrant populations, the 2 largest immigrant populations.[37] Our growth curve analysis revealed that for both Asian and Latino youth, ethnic identification and mainstream US identification changed over time. Both ethnic identification (β = −0.19, P = .002) and US identification (β = −0.13, P = .05) increased significantly from 10th to 11th grades and then declined from 11th through 12th grade. These findings are congruent with the theory that adolescence is a developmental period when youth engage in discovering their ethnic identity[21,45] early in their high school years and then stabilize into a more permanent ethnic identity during middle to later adolescence.[46,47]

The authors also explored the relations between immigrant youth's levels of US and ethnic identification and their mental health symptoms.[36] US identification was not significantly related to internalizing mental health symptoms for Asian or Latino youth, indicating that acculturation into the mainstream US culture itself does not seem to serve as a protective factor for either group. Ethnic identity, however, emerged as a protective factor. It was found that higher levels of ethnic identification were related to lower levels of withdrawn/depressed symptoms (β = −0.04, P = .04) for both Asian and Latino youth. Further, higher levels of ethnic identity also protected against somatic complaints, but this relation was moderated by ethnicity (β = 0.06, P = .05). Specifically, greater ethnic identity predicted fewer somatic complaints for Asian youth (P = .002) but not Latino youth (P = .62). These results reveal the importance of ethnic identity in mental health for immigrant populations, but they also demonstrate important differences between ethnic groups that professionals must be mindful of.

CLINICAL IMPLICATIONS

The American Psychological Association's Presidential Task Force on Immigration concluded that the field of psychology had insufficient information about the lives of a large and growing segment of North American culture: immigrants.[48] This task force also concluded that mental health clinicians, in general, lacked important knowledge, skills, and resources necessary for providing excellent services to immigrant clients.[48–50] The lack of adequate services for immigrants has contributed to underutilization across immigrant groups.[51,52] Other factors also contribute to underutilization, including language barriers, a lack of information on how to obtain services and navigate the US health care system, limited financial resources, cultural mistrust toward mental health professionals, in part due to contradictions between cultural and personal values, and values of the status quo often upheld within mental health treatment.[36,48,53]

The American Psychological Association (APA) task force on immigration found no difference in levels of mental health distress between immigrant populations and the US born population. This finding is in line with the findings of our work that youth in immigrant families are resilient and generally gravitate toward increased mental health over their development. When immigrants do seek mental health services, their distress is often directly linked to the immigration experience, such as language, cultural differences, and generational differences.[24,48,54] Importantly, recent research has also found a clear link between experiences of prejudice and discrimination in their new environment and mental health distress.[37] The total of immigration-related stresses is linked with both internalizing and externalizing coping patterns including depression, anxiety, and substance abuse/dependence.[37]

When taken together, immigrants' reasons for underutilizing treatment become clearer. Overall, as a field, we do not provide adequate services because we are not learning and training with adequate resources. Immigrants and people of color are still underrepresented in training programs. Consequently, the general demographics among service providers fail to reflect the demographics of North America. Not surprisingly, when clients experience cultural incompetence in therapy, they develop a negative view of therapy in general.[26] No client should ever experience microaggressions or stereotypes within therapy. Microaggressions in the context of therapeutic contexts are subtle and ambiguous acts committed by therapists who are unaware that they are being insensitive or discriminatory. Victims who experience microaggressions experience uncertainty and doubt about their perception of discrimination due to the ambiguous nature of microaggressions. Microaggression in therapy indicates an urgent need to improve this field's knowledge base and training approaches. There is a growing consensus that multicultural learning involves a flexibility of thought, which Jun[55] refers to as "transformative learning" or the combination of intellectual understanding and knowledge with emotional understanding or affect. Cultural competence does not require one to know everything about a client's culture at the outset, but to be proactive in their learning and humble in their lack of knowledge.[26]

Despite the gaps in our knowledge, a core aspect of cultural competence is familiarizing oneself with best practices for working with immigrant youth. The APA[48] recommends that considerations in assessment of immigrant clients include modifying testing to address language barriers. This includes using language appropriate tests, not using timed tests, or relying on alternate, less language-dependent means of assessment. If these measures are not taken, immigrant clients can be misdiagnosed, overpathologized, or their needs overlooked. Assessment must also involve consideration of cultural differences in how mental health is experienced. Disorders vary between cultures, and without enough knowledge about cultural variation, clinicians may miss important symptoms or pathologize healthy, culturally appropriate behavior.[48,56] Assessment for immigrants must include consideration of the reasons for immigrating, traumatic experiences, and losses related to immigrating, as well as the social, interpersonal experiences within the host culture.[26] Finally, clinicians should be aware of their immigrant clients' multiple cultural identities. Immigrants' mental health is protected if they keep a positive sense of belonging with their culture of origin, but they also need a healthy sense of belonging to American culture. Therapists should keep these multiple community needs in mind and be mindful of how these may differ between generations.

In summary, culturally competent therapy must involve actively seeking available knowledge about working effectively with immigrants in general and with the particular cultures of one's clients; this must involve understanding the stressors associated with acculturation and the influence these stressors can have on mental health. At the same time, clinicians must understand that the available knowledge is limited. Thus, an attitude of cultural humility and willingness to learn, in the context of a strong working alliance, is also necessary.

SUMMARY

Youth in immigrant families in the United States face growing antiimmigrant sentiment, which poses as developmental risk factors to their successful adaptation and development. The sociopolitical challenges and institutional and cultural barriers influence the acculturation experiences of immigrant youth and have negative implications for acculturative stress and mental health outcomes. Further research is needed to understand the important role context plays in shaping their experiences. Equally important is to equip our clinicians with culturally competent resources and training. Studies demonstrate that youth in immigrant families thrive and are resilient, yet, we have the responsibility to change the negative circumstances that are imposed on them.

REFERENCES

1. Migration Policy Institute. Frequently requested statistics on immigrants and immigration in the United States 2018. Available at: https://www.migrationpolicy.org/article/frequently-requested-statistics-immigrants- andimmi gration-united-states #Children. Accessed August 5, 2018.
2. García Coll C, Lamberty G, Jenkins R, et al. An integrative model for the study of developmental competencies in minority children. Child Dev 1996;67:1891–914.
3. Suárez-Orozco C, Motti-Stefanidi F, Marks A, et al. An integrative risk and resilience model for understanding the adaptation of immigrant-origin children and youth. Am Psychol 2018;73(6):781–96.
4. Marks AK, Godoy CM, García Coll C. An ecological approach to understanding immigrant child and adolescent developmental competencies. In: Gershoff ET, Mistry RS, Crosby DA, editors. Societal contexts of child development. New York: Oxford University Press; 2013. p. 75–89.
5. Oppedal B, Toppelberg C. Culture competence: a developmental task of acculturation. In: Sam DL, Berry JW, editors. The Cambridge handbook of acculturation psychology revised. Cambridge (United Kingdom): Cambridge University Press; 2016. p. 71–92.
6. Center for Immigration Studies. Immigrants in the United States: a profile of America's foreign-born population 2018. Available at: https://cis.org/Immigrants-United-States- Profile-Americas-ForeignBorn-Population. Accessed October 1, 2018.

7. Ebert K, Ovink SM. Anti-immigrant ordinances and discrimination in new and established destinations. Am Behav Sci 2014;58(13):1784–804.
8. Migration Policy Institute. U.S. Immigration policy under trump: deep changes and lasting impacts 2018. Available at: https://www.migrationpolicy.org/research/us-immigration-policy-trump-deep-changes-impacts. Accessed October 1, 2018.
9. Pew Research Center. Shifting public views on legal immigration into the U.S 2018. Available at: http://assets.pewresearch.org/wp- content/uploads/sites/5/2018/06/02164131/06-28-2018-Immigration-release.pdf.
10. Quinnipiac University. Stop taking the kids, 66 percent of U.S. Voters say, Quinnipiac University National Poll Finds; Support for dreamers is 79 percent 2018. Available at: https://poll.qu.edu/national/release-detail?ReleaseID=2550. Accessed August 5, 2018.
11. Berry J. Applied cross-Cultural psychology. 2nd edition. Cambridge (England): Cambridge University Press; 2002.
12. Redfield R, Linton R, Herskovitz M. Memorandum for the Study of Acculturation. Am Anthropol 1936;38:149–52.
13. Berry J, Trimble J, Olmedo E. Assessment of acculturation. In: Lonner WJ, Berry J, editors. Field methods in cross-cultural research. Thousand Oaks (CA): Sage Publications; 1986. p. 291–324.
14. Gordon M. Assimilation in American life: the role of race, religion and national origins. 1st edition. New York: Oxford University Press; 1964.
15. Ryder A, Alden L, Paulhus D. Is acculturation unidimensional or bidimensional? A head-to-head comparison in the prediction of personality, self-identity, and adjustment. J Pers Soc Psychol 2000;79(1):49–65.
16. Benet-Martinez V, Haritatos J. Bicultural identity integration (BII): components and psychosocial antecedents. J Pers 2005;73(4):1015–50.
17. Schwartz SJ, Zamboanga BL, Rodriguez L, et al. The structure of cultural identity in an ethnically diverse sample of emerging adults. Basic Appl Soc Psych 2007; 29(2):159–73.
18. Tadmor C, Tetlock P. A model of the effects of second-culture exposure on acculturation and integrative complexity. J Cross Cult Psychol 2006;37(2):173–90.
19. Miller MJ, Yang M, Hui K, et al. Acculturation, enculturation, and Asian American college students' mental health and attitudes toward seeking professional psychological help. J Couns Psychol 2011;58(3):346–57.
20. Berry J, Hou F. Immigrant acculturation and wellbeing in Canada. Can Psychol 2016;57(4):254–64.
21. Berry JW, Phinney JS, Sam DL, et al. Immigrant youth: acculturation, identity, and adaptation. Appl Psychol 2006;55:303–32.
22. Nguyen A, Benet-Martínez V. Biculturalism and adjustment: a meta-analysis. J Cross Cult Psychol 2013;44:122–59.
23. Behrens K, del Pozo MA, Großhennig A, et al. How much orientation towards the host culture is healthy? Acculturation style as risk enhancement for depressive symptoms in immigrants. Int J Soc Psychiatry 2015;61(5):498–505.
24. Suarez-Orozco C, Suarez-Orozco MM. Children of immigration. London: Harvard University Press; 2001.
25. Sirin SR, Ryce P. Cultural incongruence between teachers and families: implications for immigrant students. In: Takanishi R, Grigerenko, editors. Immigration, diversity, and education. London: Routledge/Taylor; 2009. p. 151–69.
26. Rogers-Sirin L, Ryce P, Sirin S. Acculturation, acculturative stress, and cultural mismatch and their influences on immigrant children and adolescents' well-being. In: Dimitrova R, Bender M, van de Vijver F, editors. Global perspectives on

well-being in immigrant families. Advances in immigrant family research. New York: Springer; 2014. p. 11–30.

27. Park W. Acculturative stress and mental health among Korean adolescents in the United States. J Hum Behav Soc Environ 2009;19(5):626–34.

28. Hwang W, Ting J. Disaggregating the effects of acculturation and acculturative stress on the mental health of Asian Americans. Cultur Divers Ethnic Minor Psychol 2008;14(2):147–54.

29. Burnett-Zeigler I, Bohnert KM, Ilgen MA. Ethnic identity, acculturation and the prevalence of lifetime psychiatric disorders among Black, Hispanic, and Asian adults in the U.S. J Psychiatr Res 2013;47(1):56–63.

30. Ng TK, Wang KC, Chan W. Acculturation and cross-cultural adaptation: the moderating role of social support. Int J Intercult Relat 2017;59:19–30.

31. Lee JS, Koeske GF, Sales E. Social support buffering of acculturative stress: a study of mental health symptoms among Korean international students. Int J Intercult Relat 2004;28(5):399–414.

32. Jibeen T. Moderators of acculturative stress in Pakistani immigrants: the role of personal and social resources. Int J Intercult Relat 2011;35(5):523–33.

33. Wei M, Liao KY-H, Heppner PP, et al. Forbearance coping, identification with heritage culture, acculturative stress, and psychological distress among chinese international students. J Couns Psychol 2012;59(1):97–106.

34. Kim E, Hogge I, Salvisberg C. Effects of self-esteem and ethnic identity: acculturative stress and psychological well-being among Mexican immigrants. Hisp J Behav Sci 2014;36(2):144–63.

35. Roley ME, Kawakami R, Baker J, et al. Family cohesion moderates the relationship between acculturative stress and depression in Japanese adolescent temporary residents. J Immigr Minor Health 2014;16(6):1299–302.

36. Rogers-Sirin L, Gupta T. Cultural identity and mental health: differing trajectories among Asian and Latino youth. J Couns Psychol 2012;59:555–66.

37. Sirin SR, Ryce R, Gupta T, et al. The role of acculturative stress on mental health symptoms for immigrant adolescents: a longitudinal investigation. Dev Psychol 2013;49(4).

38. Mena FJ, Padilla AM, Maldonado M. Acculturative stress and specific coping strategies among immigrant and later generation college students [Special issue]. Hisp J Behav Sci 1987;9:207–25.

39. Achenbach TM. Manual for the youth self-report and 1991 profile. Burlington (VT): University of Vermont Department of Psychiatry; 1991.

40. Suárez-Orozco C, Suárez-Orozco M, Todorova I. Learning a new land: immigrant students in American society. Cambridge (MA): Harvard University Press; 2008.

41. Crocker J, Luhtanen R, Blaine B, et al. Collective self-esteem and psychological well-being among White, Black, and Asian College students. Pers Soc Psychol Bull 1994;20(5):503–13.

42. Gil AG, Vega WA, Dimas JM. Acculturative stress and personal adjustment among Hispanic adolescent boys. J Community Psychol 1994;22:43–54.

43. Hovey JD. Acculturative stress, depression, and suicidal ideation in Mexican immigrants. Cultur Divers Ethnic Minor Psychol 2000;6:134–51.

44. Smokowski PR, Bacallao M. Acculturation, internalizing mental health symptoms, and self-esteem: cultural experiences of Latino adolescents in North Carolina. Child Psychiatry Hum Dev 2007;37:273–92.

45. Fuligni A. Family obligation and assistance during adolescence: contextual variations and developmental implications (new directions in child and adolescent development monograph). San Francisco (CA): Jossey-Bass, Inc; 2001. p. 61–76.

46. French SE, Seidman E, Allen L, et al. Racial/ethnic identity, congruence with the social context, and the transition to high school. J Adolesc Res 2000;15:587–602.
47. Phinney JS. The multigroup ethnic identity measure a new- scale for use with diverse groups. J Adolesc Res 1992;7:156–76.
48. American Psychological Association. Crossroads: the psychology of immigration in the new century. Report of the Presidential Taskforce on Immigration. Washington, DC: American Psychological Association; 2012.
49. Abe-Kim J, Takeuchi DT, Hong S, et al. Use of mental health-related services among immigrant and U. S.-born Asian Americans: results from the National Latino and Asian American Study. Am J Public Health 2007;97:91–8.
50. Yang LH, Worpat-Borja AJ. Psychopathology among Asian Americans. In: Leong FTL, Inman A, Ebreo A, et al, editors. Handbook of Asian American psychology. 2nd edition. Thousand Oaks (CA): Sage; 2007. p. 379–406.
51. Rivera-Mosquera E, Mitchell-Blanks M, Lopez-Garcia E, et al. The future of counseling immigrants and their families. In: Zagelbaum A, Carlson J, editors. Working with immigrant families. New York: Routledge; 2011. p. 229–60.
52. Wang L, Freeland D. Coping with immigration: new challenges for the mental health profession. In: Lau Chin J, editor. The psychology of prejudice and discrimination, volume 2: ethnicity and multiracial identity. Westport (CT): Praeger Publishers; 2009. p. 161–92.
53. David EJR. Cultural mistrust and mental health help-seeking attitudes among Filipino Americans. Asian Am J Psychol 2010;57–66. https://doi.org/10.1037/a0018814.
54. Fine M, Sirin SR. Theorizing hyphenated selves: muslim american youth negotiating identities on the fault lines of global conflict. Soc Personal Psychol Compass 2007;11(3):16–38.
55. Jun H. Social justice, multicultural counseling, and practice: beyond a convention approach. London: Sage Publications; 2010.
56. Sue DW, Sue D. Counseling the culturally diverse: theory and practice. 6th edition. Hoboken (NJ): John Wiley & Sons; 2012.

Building on Resiliencies of Refugee Families

Mary Fabio, MD[a], Lisa D. Parker, MSS[b],*, Meera B. Siddharth, MD[c]

KEYWORDS

- Resiliency • Refugee • Culturally responsive care • Pediatric care
- Trauma-informed care • Self-advocacy

KEY POINTS

- Clinicians should recognize the strengths and resiliencies of their refugee patients and build on those in the clinical relationship.
- Clinicians should be aware that the refugee experience is informed by stressors throughout the resettlement process, from the home country, to the transit country, and finally to the United States.
- Strong family bonds and a connection to community members from the same country of origin help to build resilience within refugee families.
- Clinicians play an important role in helping refugee patients navigate the complex medical system and to develop self-advocacy.

Through the world of the United Nations High Commission for Refugees—often on the front lines of conflict—we witness the courage, tenacity and brilliance of refugees every single day. Having lost their homes, their work, and sometimes their families—they don't give up—they find a way to start again. Striving to belong, and to contribute, they reach out to their new neighbors, building connections, and creating new opportunities.
—Filippo Grandi, United Nations High Commissioner for Refugees (UNHCR)[1]

According to the UNHCR, there are currently 25.4 million refugees worldwide, the highest number ever recorded.[2] Approximately half of these refugees are children under the age of 18.[2] In 2017, 102,800 refugees were resettled globally.[2] According to the State Department, 85,000 refugees were resettled in the United States in fiscal year 2016,[3] and fewer than 54,000 were admitted in fiscal year 2017.[4]

[a] Children's Hospital of Philadelphia, Karabots Pediatric Care Center, 4865 Market Street, Philadelphia, PA 19139, USA; [b] Peace Day Philly, Philadelphia, PA, USA; [c] Children's Hospital of Philadelphia, 3501 Civic Center Boulevard, Emergency Department, Colket Building, 2nd Floor, Philadelphia PA 19104, USA
* Corresponding author. P.O. Box 534, Devon, PA 19333.
E-mail address: contact@peacedayphilly.org

Pediatr Clin N Am 66 (2019) 655–667
https://doi.org/10.1016/j.pcl.2019.02.011
0031-3955/19/© 2019 Elsevier Inc. All rights reserved.

As waves of refugees have come to the United States over the years, health care practitioners have worked to provide them with adequate medical care. Pediatric clinics in Philadelphia, where 875 refugees settled in 2016,[5] have made important adjustments to better serve the linguistic, cultural, and experiential needs of refugee families. The pediatric refugee clinic at Children's Hospital of Philadelphia, along with others that have developed across the country, are models for clinics seeking to serve refugee children and their families in ways that are culturally responsive and draw upon the strengths and resiliencies of refugee families.

SCOPE OF THE ISSUE: COMMON REFUGEE EXPERIENCES

"Implicit in the refugees' experiences were states of culture shock, loneliness, psychic numbness, grief, nostalgia, and feelings of dejection, humiliation, inferiority, and feeling as if they belonged nowhere."[6]

Refugee families have experienced multiple, significant stressors and/or traumas by the time they present at US pediatric clinics.[7,8] These stressors and traumas can include persecution and violence in their home country. For example, members can be injured, killed, or separated from the family in the midst of their country's conflict. Children may have seen family members abused or killed, or may have witnessed the destruction of their home and belongings.

Refugee families have also experienced stressors during the migration journey, including living in a state of uncertainty for years in refugee camps or transient areas within other countries.[7,8] As a result of this uncertainty, most refugee families live with the anxiety of having no sense of when, where, or if they are going to be resettled. Traumatic experiences, such as physical abuse or witnessing violence, are also not uncommon in refugee camps.[9]

Refugee camps/transient areas have differing levels of pediatric health care. Generally, however, these environments have limited educational and health care supports. Common health issues of refugee children upon arrival to the United States include dental and optometry needs, low weight, chronic hepatitis B, latent tuberculosis, parasitic infections, high blood lead levels, and anemia. The refugee population is also more likely to have preexisting health problems than other immigrants because of the stressors of migration.[10]

Once in the United States, refugees experience an additional set of stressors that relate to the process of adapting to a completely new society- structurally, linguistically and culturally. For example, most refugees live in poverty when they are resettled in the United States,[11] and this can result in a significant sense of disillusionment. A less-empowered status impacts the ability of refugees to "re-establish place, re-structure identity, and regain a sense of belonging."[12] As a result, refugees often need to adjust expectations in alignment with the realities of their new lives. According to Nadège U. Mukamusoni of the Nationalities Service Center, "The refugee resettlement transition isn't an easy process; if refugees had a choice, they would stay in their home countries."[13]

Language and system barriers can make it difficult for refugee families to adapt to their new environment and to effectively seek help. Refugees from the same country of origin may not speak the same language, and refugee families who prefer rare languages may be at particular risk for linguistic and cultural isolation.[14] Isolation and limited opportunities to interact with families of their own culture, due to refugee families living in different parts of a city, can be additional significant factors impeding successful resettlement.

Refugee families arriving in the United States are eligible for support from resettlement agencies for only 90 days. These agencies assist with essential housing, school, employment, social services, mental health and physical health needs and play a critical role in the process of refugee adaptation to the United States and eventual self-advocacy. Agencies can also assist families in accessing multiple health care systems, particularly in cases of complex medical conditions.

Physical, mental, and emotional stressors of resettled refugee families, in addition to language barriers, can include undertreated chronic health conditions; socioeconomic issues; values conflict/cultural bereavement; racism/discrimination; and mental health issues. Rates of posttraumatic stress disorder can reach 86% in the refugee population.[14] These rates compare with 6.8% of the general US population. Racial discrimination can also be a challenge to psychological and cultural resettlement. People born in countries where English is not the primary language are much more likely to experience discrimination related to education, housing, workplace, community, and policing. Discrimination can compound already existent stressors and contribute to acculturation stress.[15]

Individual and family adjustments to the challenging combination of resettlement issues, in addition to effectively managing the traumas and losses experienced during their refugee journey, are critical for positive health outcomes. In a systematic review of individual, family, community, and societal risk and protective factors, multiple factors impact child and adolescent mental health after resettlement.[7] Protective factors include family cohesion and strong parental support, a safe school system, peer support, and a welcoming community in country of resettlement. The pediatrician can play an important role in positive sociocultural adaptation through encouraging family cohesion and parental support as well as in helping families to access positive educational and community resources.

The ability of refugee families to interface successfully within US health care, educational, and social service systems may at times be negatively impacted by the complexity and lack of coordination of some of these systems.[16] Clinicians can play a critical role in helping refugee families successfully navigate imperfect systems of pediatric care (**Fig. 1**).

RESILIENCE

Refugees who arrive in the United States are resilient. They have fled conflict, survived insecurity in a neighboring country, made it to our shores with smiles intact and navigated the resettlement process. Our job is to continue to foster that resilience as they resettle in our communities by supporting their integration. Our mandate as pediatricians is to advocate for and nurture children and their families so that they can maintain good health, heal old wounds and thrive in their new country.[17]

Despite a myriad of stressors and, in some cases, multiple traumas, refugee families consistently demonstrate both individual and family strengths and resiliencies. On the whole, refugees have had to develop positive internal and familial strengths in order to adapt and survive. Furthermore, and despite many barriers, refugees are frequently able to create a sense of stability in their families and become positive contributors to society.[18] These strengths and accomplishments can be reinforce in part through the clinician-patient/family relationship as well as resettlement agency involvement.

Resilience is defined as "the capacity to recover quickly from difficulties; toughness." Those with resilience have innate characteristics that include strength,

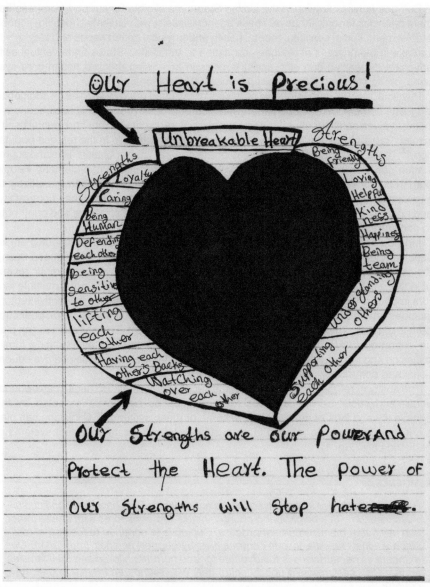

Fig. 1. Drawing by a young Somali woman who came to the United States as a refugee when she was a teenager. She now has children of her own. In this drawing, she identifies the strengths in her community, which have helped her family succeed in this country.

adaptability, belonging, and purpose. Resilience has also been defined as "the capacity of a dynamic system (individual, family, school, community, society) to withstand or recover from significant challenges that threaten its stability, viability, or development."[19] Furthermore, resilience is an ongoing process rather than a fixed personal quality.[20] Resilience can also be defined "as a dynamic process that shifts in response to new vulnerabilities and adversities."[21]

Resilience with regard to refugees relates to internal psychological strength as well as creation of external familial, ethnic, cultural, and environmental supports. Access to religious and spiritual settings can also play an important role in refugee family resilience.[22] In addition, according to the UNHCR's Senior Mental Health Officer Pieter Ventevogel, "Some of the most powerful mental health interventions are not medical, but are related to empowering people and strengthening support within refugee communities."[23]

Positive emotions in refugee families, such as relief from the threat of death in their old home and the opportunity to create permanence and normalcy in their lives, are factors that can aid in successful adaptation.[24] Characteristics such as optimism, adaptability, and perseverance, also positively relate to refugee resilience.[25] Tapping into these emotions during the clinic appointment can be a key to creating a trusting relationship and a sense of empowerment on the part of the parents and/or older children. Clinicians need to honor refugees' "capacity for resilience" and "foster positive adaptation by helping them obtain and protect internal and environmental resources."[24]

CULTURALLY RESPONSIVE CARE

We are often so focused on documenting the negative aspects of war. But that is only half the story. We found that [youth who are refugees] actually prefer that you focus on their strengths rather than their vulnerabilities, their dignity rather than their misery, their capacity rather than their vulnerability, and their resources and their agency rather than their victimhood.
— Catherine Panter-Brick, anthropologist[26]

The American Academy of Pediatrics (AAP) regards the "vital and critical value" of providing culturally effective pediatric care. The Institute of Medicine defines patient-centered care as "care that is respectful of and responsive to individual patient preferences, needs, and values."[27] The focus of health care delivery should include developing strategies that improve the delivery of culturally effective care as well as addressing barriers to effective health care.[28]

Federal law requires that health care providers receiving federal funding offer appropriate language services for patients with limited English proficiency. Language barriers can result in confusing communication in terms of medical questions and directives; moreover, they can negatively impact rapport and can increase medical errors.[29] Working effectively with interpreters greatly aids the identification of family strengths, as well as areas of risk, within the clinic setting.

Although the need for accurate interpreting is a critical component of care, there are number of other important components of a culturally responsive refugee pediatric health clinic. For example, the quality of communication and patient-provider interaction, including empathy shown by providers, can have a powerful impact on treatment adherence as well as seeking out future health care.[30] In addition, a strengths-based versus deficits-based approach allows practitioners to help refugee families build on existing resiliencies.[22]

Practitioners should be mindful of the many issues and challenges that refugee families may have faced, while at the same time identifying and building on strengths and positive strides in the course of the clinical interaction. When practitioners express genuine interest in and curiosity about refugee family experiences, rather than making assumptions, the clinician-family relationship is enhanced. Being open to hearing about a family's refugee journey, without pressing, can be an important step in building trust.

Practitioner "self-reflection, self-knowledge, and self-critique" are necessary in order to be effective in communicating with people of different cultures.[28] In addition, clinician training programs should focus on honing interpersonal skills to nurture clinician-patient relationships, including with patient groups of differing cultures. Doing so positively impacts both the resiliency and the health status of patients.

Tools such as the AAP's, Immigrant Child Health Toolkit and "Trauma Informed," a Trauma Toolkit, can support clinicians in understanding health, cultural, and trauma issues relevant to refugee populations.[31] These toolkits offer information about important topics, such as approaching care from a strengths-based perspective; implementing clinic accommodations; how to speak sensitively with people who have experienced trauma; and clinical interactions that keep in mind possible mental health considerations. This information can be very valuable in terms of helping pediatricians develop approaches based on best practices, and as a result more effectively support greater resilience in the families they serve.

It can be very effective for the development of a positive relationship that, whenever possible, clinicians connect with refugees through community-based activities, such as community-based health fairs.[32] "Medicine is just the tip of the iceberg. The tentacles out to the community are key. Parents bring unique perspectives that deepen our understanding of the refugee experience. Hearing their stories helps us connect with our patients on a human level and improves the care we provide."[33]

CASE STUDIES

The 3 following cases illustrate the resilience of refugee families. Each case also highlights compassionate, strengths-based provider-patient/family interactions that encourage the development of independence and self-advocacy (**Fig. 2**).

Case 1

Manal is an 8-year-old girl from Iraq. Her family of 5 fled the war to Jordan when she was 6 years old. While in the refugee camp in Jordan, Manal had recurrent nightmares from her traumatic experiences in Iraq. The family's home town in Iraq was frequently subjected to bomb blasts, and many neighborhood homes were destroyed. In addition, one day, Iraqi soldiers forced their way in to their home while her dad was away. They searched the home and destroyed all of the children's toys. As a result of these traumatic experiences, Manal panicked and ran to her parents with every loud noise. In addition, she hid all of her toys in her closet as soon as she was done playing with them.

Upon arrival to the United States, Manal's parents expressed concerns about her behaviors. She refused to sleep in her own bed and continued to have nightmares. The parents used management strategies that we discussed at the initial and follow-up visits. They were counseled about sleep routines, the importance of reassurance, managing her anxiety and stress, and focusing on school enrollment and resettlement goals. Once given tools, the family was able to implement these suggestions, and by the next visit 2 months later, Manal was sleeping in her own bed.

The parents independently sought support from the local Iraqi community. Interacting with other community members who had been through similar trauma and had resettled successfully encouraged Manal's family. These community connections helped the entire family feel more comfortable and accepted in their new home.

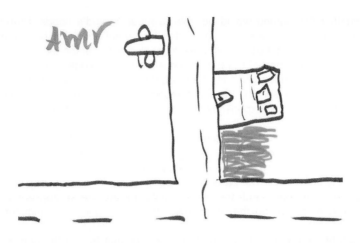

Fig. 2. When asked to describe his life in Syria, a 10-year-old boy drew planes flying over his house, dropping chemicals.

This case clearly demonstrates how important it is to use the existing strengths of each family. All members of the family had been traumatized in their home country. The parents, despite trauma, had the resilience to access internal, relational, and community strengths to manage their negative experiences and emotions. Through their close family bonds and willingness to learn and use additional coping strategies, the parents effectively helped their children manage and overcome their anxiety. The father is now working as a medical interpreter, and all three children are thriving emotionally and academically.

Case 2

Ahmed G. is a 13-year-old Syrian refugee who arrived to the United States three years ago after spending four years in Iraq. Ahmed was previously diagnosed with autism and had attended an autism support school in Syria for five years. During the four years his family spent in Iraq, Ahmed was unable to attend school. His mother spent all her time with him, because his behavior was difficult to control and she needed to be by his side at all times.

In his first encounter for his domestic medical examination, Ahmed was nonverbal but was able to communicate and express emotions, had several facial tics, and was very impulsive and erratic in his behaviors. Ahmed was unable to sit still in the room, so his mother walked him through the hallways of the office while his father spoke to the doctor. His father reported that a psychiatrist in Jordan had recommended that Ahmed take risperidone to calm him down for the plane trip to the United States. Unfortunately, Ahmed had a paradoxical reaction to the medication, and they had a very difficult journey. His father believed that the combination of the risperidone and the journey had exacerbated Ahmed's erratic behavior.

Although Ahmed's siblings were enrolled in school within a week of arrival, Ahmed's family had to enroll him in a school further from their home because it had an autism support classroom. Familiar with the school, the pediatrician had some reservations about whether this setting would be able to meet Ahmed's needs. Unfortunately, because he had never been seen by a developmental specialist or psychiatrist in the United States, the school did not have a detailed report of the extent of his needs. The school district informed the father that Ahmed was obliged to try to go to this school, and if it was not a good fit, they would then address the issue. However, at Ahmed's first day of school, he experienced overstimulation, leading him to be restrained. This traumatic experience for Ahmed led his parents to keep him home after that day.

The pediatrician worked with the resettlement agency and the family to advocate for Ahmed with the school district. During this process, the parents were dismayed when they received a truancy notice, because Ahmed had missed more school days than the law allows. The parents managed to remain hopeful despite the irony of the situation: on one hand, the school could not provide an appropriate school setting for Ahmed, but on the other hand, they were penalizing him for missing school.

Ahmed's father continued to push the school district to find the right school for him. After visiting a few schools, they finally agreed on a private school an hour away, which was paid for by the school district. At this point, his father had learned quite a bit about the educational rights for his child. He was later hired by the school district as an Arabic interpreter for families that were in similar situations as his family.

Although the US educational system can be difficult to navigate, especially for families with a child who has special needs, Ahmed's family experienced additional roadblocks, including delayed evaluation and provision of services. This family persisted and was able to overcome the barriers unique to their special situation.

This case demonstrates that with some direction from the provider, the inherent strengths of this family enabled them to successfully navigate the complex educational system and successfully advocate for the special educational needs of their child.

Case 3

A new family from a refugee camp in Uganda came into the clinic. The family consisted of the matriarch, Patience, and four children, aged 15, 13, and 10 years old and a 15-month-old toddler. As the story of their migration journey unfolded, Patience revealed that the toddler, Mariama, was the child of her 15-year-old daughter, Faith. It was disclosed that Mariama was the product of a rape in the refugee camp in Uganda. Faith was attacked while foraging for food on the outskirts of the camp, an all too familiar story. During this initial visit in refugee clinic, Faith deferred to her mother to speak about the care of Mariama. When Mariama received shots, she went to her grandmother, Patience, for comfort.

The family continued to receive care in the refugee clinic. At every visit, an effort was made to address Faith, not Faith's her mother, about the physical and emotional needs of Mariama. Faith was encouraged to read to Mariama daily. Providers offered books provided through the Reach Out and Read Program[34] and discussed how to look at books and talk about the pictures with Mariama, even if Faith was unable to read the words due to her limited literacy. Patience also encouraged Faith to assume the role of primary caretaker for Mariama. In time, Faith seemed to be adjusting well, attending high school, learning English, and caring lovingly for Mariama.

At her yearly checkup, Faith came in obviously expecting a baby. She had not yet had any prenatal care. When told that her pregnancy test was positive, Faith disclosed that she had been raped by an older man. During the clinical encounter, the initial telephonic interpreter was a man. Faith was very uncomfortable with this discussion through a male interpreter. The interpreter agency was contacted, and a female interpreter was located to help Faith tell her story more easily.

Faith needed to feel supported in order to trust her care providers. Faith was able to urgently have an ultrasound and see an obstetrician. Her pediatrician maintained close contact with Faith and her mother after visits to make sure they were doing well and understood all the prenatal and newborn instructions. During discussions about caring for a new baby, the pediatrician identified the need for education and practical assistance with meeting "Back to Sleep" recommendations.[35] The office social worker became involved and contacted a nonprofit group to provide Faith with a bassinet, bedding for a baby, and many other necessary items. These items were delivered to Faith's home by the refugee clinic provider, who visited the home and helped set them up.

In an effort to recover from her multiple traumas, Faith joined a youth group at a local church serving the refugee community. There she was able to interact with peers, which helped decrease her isolation. She participated in important educational activities focusing on navigating public transportation and sex education. Accessing these supports enhanced her ability to attend school and care for her children.

The combination of parental, clinician, and sociocultural support enabled Faith, with her foundation of loving care for her children, to overcome multiple traumas and develop self-advocacy. This case also emphasizes the need for clear, respectful, and compassionate communication and appropriate interpretation. The provider focused on medical needs but also identified nonmedical issues that needed to be resolved and helped to support those needs.

CLINICAL RECOMMENDATIONS

People often talk about refugees as victims, as people to be pitied, and surely they have experienced much more than their fair share of pain, loss and heartache in their lives. But refugees are also among the most resilient people that I've ever met. They made it here for one! The U.S. resettles just 1% of refugees in need of resettlement and these folks are among the few that get that chance. They are survivors. And while the US resettlement experience is incredibly hard, they are laser-focused on making it work.[36]

Based on the available evidence base and the authors' clinical experiences, the following are suggestions with regard to providing culturally responsive, strengths-based care to refugee families:

1. Identify the families' areas of strength/resiliency and build on these.
2. Provide a dedicated refugee clinic where patients can be seen by the same providers.
3. Schedule extra time for the first 3 to 4 clinic visits with refugee families to allow for time to build a relationship and to work through an interpreter.
4. Ensure appropriate interpreting resources for families within the health care setting.
5. When using an interpreter, look at the family while speaking and share only 1 to 2 sentences at a time. Assess accuracy of interpretation in an ongoing way.
6. Make a point to understand the pronunciation of the child's first and last name; consider including phonetic pronunciation of names in the chart.
7. Use available online resources for translated pediatric medical information. These include "Health Information Translations": http://bit.ly/2kh55HB.

8. Recognize conditions, such as infectious diseases, not commonly found in US patients, and be aware of particular health issues, such as high levels of lead within children from Afghanistan or vitamin D deficiency among girls who wear a hijab.[37] For more information, research "Refugee Health Profiles": https://www.cdc.gov/immigrantrefugeehealth/profiles/index.html.
8. For inpatient situations, coordinate with social workers and outside agencies before discharge to optimize transition from hospital to home, including ensuring that basic needs impacting infant/child health can be met.
9. Welcome refugee families with patience and compassion. Acknowledge their difficult journeys and be open to hearing their stories.
10. Demonstrate sensitivity and compassion regarding possible past physical and emotional trauma as well as the stress of transition to a new culture.
11. Learn about the families' values and practices as a means of providing culturally responsive care.
12. When encouraging a health behavior, check to see if this is something the family can do within their belief system.
13. Assess clinic paperwork for possible adjustments/translations and take note of/modify paperwork that is confusing to families.
14. Work closely with resettlement agencies. Through these agencies, refugees can receive critical nonmedical support during their first 3 months in the United States.
15. Foster self-advocacy with regard to accessing health care systems and community resources.
16. Train staff and residents in working effectively with people from different cultures.
17. Connect the family with social work and, when indicated, mental health supports beyond the 90-day period within which refugee resettlement organizations are involved. Social service supports, such as The Philadelphia Partnership for Resilience,[38] that works with survivors of torture and their families in the greater Philadelphia region, can be valuable resources.
18. Connect families with community programs where they can interact with refugee families from their home countries.
19. Be visible in refugee communities by offering free or low-cost services in collaboration with an organization that is trusted by the refugee community.
20. Meet with health care practitioners at different refugee clinics to share best practices, combine research efforts, and discover the most effective approaches.

SUMMARY

Refugees come to the United States with many diverse and complex needs as well as a foundation of resiliency. Approaching refugee families within the pediatric clinic environment with openness, respect, and a resilience-building approach can support the ability of refugee children and their parents or caregivers to effectively access Western health care systems as well as other systems vital for healthy resettlement. These efforts also help build the clinician-patient relationship and adherence, which in turn improves health outcomes. Health care providers play a significant role in the resettlement process when they provide services and guidance that are both culturally sensitive and trauma informed. Key goals for working with refugee families are to build on their resiliencies and to guide them toward self-advocacy. Pediatricians serving refugee populations should familiarize themselves with the concept of resilience in the process of creating or enhancing culturally responsive clinics (**Fig. 3**).

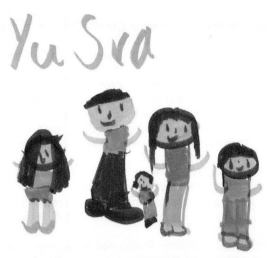

Fig. 3. When asked to describe her life in the United States, an 8-year-old girl drew a picture of her family, with her parents and the new baby, who was born after they arrived in the United States.

REFERENCES

1. UNHCR. On world refugee day, UNHCR says refugees deserve praise for resilience and courage 2017. Available at: https://bit.ly/2HFnyYx.
2. UNHCR. Global Trends: Forced displacement in 2017. Available at: https://www.unhcr.org/en-us/statistics/unhcrstats/5b27be547/unhcr-global-trends-201 7.html. Accessed January 8, 2019.
3. U.S. Department of State. Fact sheet: Fiscal year 2016 refugee admissions. Available at: https://www.state.gov/j/prm/releases/factsheets/2017/266365.htm. Accessed January 8, 2018.
4. Migration Policy Institute. Top 10 of 2017. Available at: https://www.migrationpolicy.org/article/top-10-2017-issue-6-wake-cuts-us-refugee-program-global-resettlement-falls-short. Accessed January 8, 2019.
5. Benshoff L. In 2017, PA Resettled Nearly 1,000 Fewer Refugees than the Previous Budget Year. Radio Times 2017.
6. Keyes EF, Kane CF. Belonging and adapting: mental Health of Bosnian Refugees Living in the United States. Issues Ment Health Nurs 2004;25(8):809–31.
7. Fazel M, Stein A. Mental health of displaced and refugee children resettled in high-income countries: risk and protective factors. Lancet 2012;379:266–82.
8. Lustig SL, Kia-Keating M, Grant-Knight W, et al. Review of child and adolescent refugee mental health. J Am Acad Child Adolesc Psychiatry 2004;43(1):24–36.
9. White Paper from the National Child Traumatic Stress Network Refugee Trauma Task Force. Available at: https://www.nctsn.org/sites/default/files/resources//review_child_adolescent_refugee_ mental_health.pdf. Accessed January 8, 2018.
10. Seery T, Boswell H, Lara A. Caring for refugee children. Pediatr Rev 2015;36(8):323–40.
11. Hooper K, Zong J, Capps R, et al. Young children of refugees in the United States: integration successes and challenges. Washington, DC: Migration Policy Institute; 2016. Available at: https://migrationpolicy.org/research/young-children-refugees-united-states-integration- successes-and-challenges. Accessed January 9, 2019.

12. Refugee Health Technical Assistance Center. Dynamic processes of being a refugee 2011. Available at: https://bit.ly/2ThgQKk.
13. Nadège U. Mukamusoni, case manager. Nationalities Service Center - Interview with Meera Siddharth; 2018.
14. Bolton E. PTSD in refugees. National Center for PTSD; 2016.
15. A VicHealth Survey. Ethnic and race based discrimination as a determinant of mental health and wellbeing. Available at: https://bit.ly/2JlmFqx.
16. Antonelli RC, McGallister JWM, Popp J. Making care coordination a critical component of the pediatric health system: a multidisciplinary framework. The Commonwealth Fund; 2009.
17. Andrea Green, MDCM, FAAP, Director Pediatric new American Clinic, UVM Children's Hospital Pediatric Primary Care. Interview with Lisa Parker July 2018.
18. Kerwin D. The US refugee resettlement program - a return to first principles: how refugees help to define, strengthen, and revitalize the United States. J Migr Hum Secur 2018;6(3):205–25.
19. Masten AS. Resilience in Children Threatened by Extreme Adversity: Frameworks for research, practice, and translational synergy. Dev Psychopathol 2011;23:493–506.
20. Pulvirenti M, Mason G. Resilience and survival: refugee women and violence. Curr Issues Crim Justice 2011;23(1):37–52.
21. Mohaupt S. Review article: resilience and social inclusion. Soc Policy Soc 2008;8(1):63–71.
22. Hutchinson M, Dorsett P. What does the literature say about resilience in refugee people? Implications for practice. Journal of Social Inclusion 2012;3(2):56–78.
23. Gaynor T. Q&A: Far From Being Traumatized, Most Refugees are 'Surprisingly Resilient'. UNHCR; 2017.
24. Refugee Health Technical Assistance Center - Resilience and Coping. Available at: https://bit.ly/2Hyml62.
25. Brough M, Gorman D, Ramirez E, et al. Young refugees talk about well-being: a qualitative analysis of refugee youth mental health from three states. Aust J Soc Issues 2003;38(2):193–208.
26. Singh M. How do refugee teens build resilience? NPR; 2017.
27. Frampton SB, Guastello S, Lepore M. Compassion as a Foundation of patient-centered care: the importance of compassion in action. J Comp Eff Res 2013;2(5):443–55.
28. Britton CV, American Academy of Pediatrics Committee on Pediatric Workforce. Ensuring culturally effective pediatric care: implications for education and health policy. Pediatrics 2004;114(6):1677–85.
29. Divi C, Koss RG, Loeb JM. Language Proficiency and adverse events in US hospitals: a pilot study. Int J Qual Health Care 2007;19(2):60–7.
30. Ngo-Metzger Q, Telfair J, Sorkin DH, et al. Cultural competency and quality of care: obtaining the patients perspective. The Commonwealth Fund; 2006.
31. American Academy of Pediatrics Immigrant Child Health Toolkit July 2018. Available at: https://bit.ly/2NN9cVA. Accessed June 13, 2018.
32. Sorn R, Director of Immigrant Affairs and Language Access Services, Department of Behavioral Health and disAbility Services - Interview with Lisa Parker, June 2018.
33. Andrea Shaw, MD, Assistant Professor of Pediatrics, Refugee Clinic of Upstate University Pediatric and Adolescent Center. Interview with Lisa Parker, May 2018.
34. Reach Out and Read program. Available at: http://www.reachoutandread.org/. November 10, 2018.

35. American Academy of Pediatrics Announces New Safe Sleep Recommendations to Protect Against SIDS, Sleep-Related Infant Deaths. American Academy of Pediatrics; 2016.
36. Rona Buchalter, Executive Director, HIAS-PA - Interview with Mary Fabio, June 2018.
37. Mack L. How one pediatric refugee clinic helps children move beyond the trauma. WNPR Studio 360; 2017.
38. The Philadelphia Partnership for Resilience (PPR). Available at: https://nscphila.org/ppr. November 10, 2018.

Overcoming Communication Barriers in Refugee Health Care

Sarah K. Clarke, MSPH[a],*, Janice Jaffe, PhD, CMI[b],
Raewyn Mutch, MBChB, DipRACOG, FRACP, PhD[c]

KEYWORDS

- Medical interpreters • LEP Best practice • Ethical dilemmas
- Cross-cultural communication • Culturally relevant care • Medical training

KEY POINTS

- An interpreter is a communication professional trained to interpret everything that is said, maintain confidentiality, ensure transparency, and point out cultural differences that impede communication.
- Research emphasizes the importance of working with qualified interpreters, but there is a lack of consistency in ensuring providers' training to communicate through interpreters.
- Before an encounter, providers should ensure patient interpretation preferences are met, prepare the interpreter about the visit, and practice cultural humility.
- Providers should be mindful of physical space arrangements, their speech manner and content, check in regularly with all parties during the encounter, and debrief with them after.
- Challenges (eg, logistical issues, vicarious traumatization, rare languages) can be overcome through preparation, partnerships, and flexibility.

INTRODUCTION

An abundant body of research demonstrates that language and cultural barriers negatively affect care for the estimated 9% of the population or more than 21 million people who have limited English proficiency (LEP), resulting in reduced access, higher hospitalization rates, increased risk of permanent damage, and limited health knowledge

Disclosure Statement: N/A.
[a] Society of Refugee Healthcare Providers, Spencerport, NY, USA; [b] Maine Medical Center, Hispanic Studies, Department of Romance Languages and Literatures, Bowdoin College, 7800 College Station, Brunswick, ME 04011, USA; [c] Refugee Health and General Paediatrics, Department of General Paediatrics, Perth Children's Hospital, School of Medicine, Dentistry and Health Sciences, University of Western Australia, Locked Bag 2010, 15 Hospital Avenue, Nedlands, Perth, Western Australia 6909, Australia
* Corresponding author. 134 Douglas Glen Park Southeast, Calgary, Alberta T2Z 3Z3, Canada.
E-mail address: sarahkathleen821@gmail.com

from communication difficulties.[1-5] This inequitable care proves costly: an estimated $1.24 trillion in the United States over 4 years for racial health inequalities.[6]

Culturally and Linguistically Appropriate Services for Interpreters and Providers

The need for qualified medical interpreters to mitigate these disparities is well documented.[7-10] However, qualified interpreters are only one-third of the equation when considering optimizing communication in the LEP patient-interpreter-provider triad. The National Standards for Culturally and Linguistically Appropriate Services (CLAS), developed by the US Department of Health and Human Services Office of Minority Health, present 15 action steps to guide health providers in establishing culturally and linguistically appropriate services. These steps stress that language services (interpreters) be competent, but what is missing is an action step ensuring clinicians' preparedness to work with the language service providers.[11] Similarly, the National Council on Interpreting in Health Care used national consensus-building with input from hundreds of health care interpreters to develop standards of practice and code of ethics for interpreters, but clear consensus on provider education for working with those interpreters is more difficult to find.[12-14]

Getting By

Despite high costs of health disparities for patients with LEP, legal and ethical obligations to work with qualified interpreters, and consistent correlation between effective interpreter use and improved health communication and outcomes, a 2004 national survey of United States medical residents found that 35% received little or no instruction about working through interpreters.[8,15-17] Counter to National Standards for CLAS, 84% indicated that they relied on patients' family and friends to interpret, and 22% admitted to using children, including in emergency departments and pediatrics.[11,15] Within pediatric care the improvement from 2004 to 2010 was only modest, with only 43% of pediatricians working through professional interpreters and 57% still communicating through bilingual family members.[18] A survey of pediatric residents in 2010 showed that 54% had never attended training sessions on working with professional interpreters.[19] Notably, lack of training for providers in how to access or work with interpreters is cited as a primary reason for underuse of qualified interpreters, together with underestimation of the risks of using ad hoc interpreters or family members, convenience, and a practice environment in which "getting by" is the norm.[13,19-21]

Status of Culturally Effective Care

Although the Accreditation Council for Graduate Medical Education core competencies include communication across a wide range of cultural backgrounds, and American Academy of Pediatrics (AAP) guidelines emphasize "culturally effective" care, research shows that approaches to cultural competency in medical schools and in residency programs vary dramatically, and training on communicating through interpreters with patients with LEP may be absent from clinical rotations and residency programs where they could be most beneficial.[19,22-26] On a positive note, medical students and residents express a desire for increasing their knowledge and skill in this area, and recent research has detailed successful pilot programs.[16,19,21,22,27,28]

DISCUSSION
Terminology: Interpreter Versus Translator

The terms "interpreter" and "translator" are often incorrectly used interchangeably **(Table 1)**. However, they demand significantly different training and skill sets. A

Table 1	
The difference between interpreters and translators	
Interpreter	Specialist in converting oral information from one language to another
Translator	Specialist in converting written information from one language to another
Why does it matter?	Different specialties, different skills required—it is important to know which skill is needed

translator converts written information from one language to another; an interpreter is a specialist in converting oral information from one language to another.[29] This article focuses on best practice in working with qualified interpreters. Some variation exists in different fields' requirements of interpreters, with strict rules against clarifying or considering culture in the adversarial atmosphere of a court setting.[30] In community interpreting, which includes medical interpreting, an interpreter may intervene to promote communication across cultural differences, including clarifying in cases of barriers to understanding. National certification for medical interpreters has sought to standardize interpreting practices in a rapidly evolving field, yet the degree to which interpreters may mediate to overcome cultural barriers to communication is still debated.[31–36]

Who Can and Cannot Be an Interpreter?

Persons who have demonstrated fluency in English and another language, and have successfully completed medical or health care interpretation training, can become health care interpreters (**Box 1**). This pool could include on-site interpreters, contracted interpreters (in-person, telephonic, video), trained volunteers, or bilingual health staff who satisfy the aforementioned criteria.[37] Those who cannot be an interpreter are those untrained to be an interpreter such as untrained health staff or volunteers, other patients, or visitors (**Fig. 1**). Speaking the same language is not sufficient to ensure accurate and skillful interpretation, nor does it guarantee fluency, which must be proven through testing when becoming a qualified interpreter. Patients' family members should also not be interpreters—especially and without exception, children under 18 years of age—or friends or community members.[26]

For patients with LEP, receiving care from providers who speak their language is closely correlated with improved health education, increased patient satisfaction, better health outcomes, and reduced costs and disparities.[2,38–42] However, whereas clear language proficiency requirements exist for qualified interpreters, a 2009 study reported that only 18% of hospitals with bilingual providers offered any assessment of their language proficiency, and only half of those required assessment of bilingual

Box 1	
The role of an interpreter	

An interpreter is a communication professional who is trained to:

- Interpret *everything* that is said, in first person exactly as it is said (even if it is negative or seemingly nonsensical)
- Maintain confidentiality
- Ensure transparency
- Point out cultural differences when they impede effective communication[31]

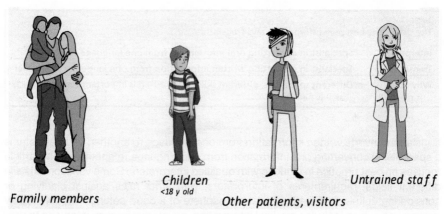

Family members   *Children*   *Other patients, visitors*   *Untrained staff*
 <18 y old

Fig. 1. Who cannot be an interpreter? (*From* "How to use interpreters effectively." Available at: https://www.youtube.com/watch?v=flB3DLEOsmg. Accessed August 24, 2018.)

physicians and nurses, thereby creating a climate in which error and miscommunication can be common.[43] Even determining the proficiency level a bilingual provider needs for adequate, safe, and effective communication with patients continues to be a challenge.[18,20,39,41,44] When self-reporting in the absence of testing, physicians tend to overestimate their language competency in another language, although some also underestimate proficiency, demonstrating the importance of reliable, formal assessment for providers to work without an interpreter.[39,44] Kaiser Permanente has instituted a formal assessment that examines both linguistic and cultural proficiency to determine whether providers may offer language-concordant care.[45] In addition, Maul and colleagues have adapted the Healthcare Failure Mode and Effects Analysis method to develop a risk-assessment approach to assist partially bilingual providers in determining when it would be prudent to request a qualified interpreter. All providers and staff should be encouraged to use their second-language skills to introduce themselves to patients and establish rapport; however, all should also work with qualified interpreters unless they have demonstrated sufficient linguistic and cultural proficiency through formal, impartial assessment.

Reimbursement (or Lack Thereof) for Interpreters

Throughout this article are references to contacting both the "insurance company" and the "language contracting company" to attempt to encompass the varied reimbursement situations in each state. A first step to working effectively with interpreters is to learn about individual states' reimbursement policies regarding interpretation and how this applies to local entities such as the managed care organizations and clinics.

Health care providers who receive federal funding are required by federal laws and guidelines to provide language access for patients with LEP,[46] but cost is often cited as a barrier for why providers are unable to provide language services.[10,47] Although states are not required to reimburse providers, federal funding does exist to assist states and health care providers with partial reimbursement (ranging from 50% to 86%) of the language services costs for those patients in the Medicaid and State Children's Health Insurance Program.[10,46] The complexity and difficulties of accessing this reimbursement vary by state, as each state structures the reimbursement differently, with many states folding language services costs into an organization's (eg, hospital, managed care organization, or clinic) administrative costs.[46] In 2007, 12 states were reported as offering direct reimbursement to providers for language services,[47] whereas other states did not offer reimbursement because of lack of awareness by policymakers about the federal funds, tight state budgets, and the belief that language services should simply be part of providers' business costs.[46] However, the National Health Law Program and The Access Project note in their report: "…but a state could allow all providers to submit for reimbursement."[46] Medicare and many private insurers, on the other hand, do not reimburse providers or states for interpretation services.[4]

Best Practice in Working with Interpreters

Although literature evaluating work with medical interpreters highlights challenges, there are generally accepted best practice tips (**Table 2**) endorsed by knowledgable organizations such as the Refugee Health Technical Assistance Center, the Gulf Coast Jewish Family and Community Services' National Partnership for Community Services, and Caring for Kids New to Canada.[7,29,48,49] These tips are meant to be used with qualified interpreters. Although some tips may take time to enact, providers may find that they ultimately save time by avoiding common issues that could occur. Also, these tips do not necessarily need to be implemented by a sole provider during any one interpreted encounter with a patient, but could be implemented by different team members.

Pre-encounter

Time available for the pre-encounter will depend on whether it is an established appointment, or an emergency or same-day consult. With even the most emergent situations, truncated versions of the pre-work (see **Table 2**) can be implemented by the provider or the clinical team.

An interpreter is a communication professional. Medical providers should follow the interpreter's guidance but also respectfully point out to the interpreter if they are not fulfilling their role in supporting communicative autonomy. Of particular importance is preparing the interpreter if the provider expects the topic to be particularly emotional or difficult. In addition, it can be helpful to plan for how the interpreter can notify the provider during the appointment if the conversation becomes too much for the patient or interpreter. If the appointment is scheduled in advance, the provider can share with the interpreter a list of medical words/questions ahead of time. Trained medical interpreters may know the vocabulary already, but this is particularly useful for specialized appointments or rare conditions. When working with telephonic interpreters, additional considerations are helpful (**Box 2**).

During the encounter

During the encounter, several considerations can facilitate optimal communication (see **Tables 2** and **4**). For instance, how the patient, health care providers, and interpreter are physically arranged can positively or negatively influence communication (**Table 3**).[50] Additionally it is critical to avoid generalizations about patients' health practices or beliefs based on their race, ethnicity, or culture. Instead, providers can ask the patient what she or he thinks the problem is, what is causing it, and how it would be treated back home (and how she/he thinks it should be treated).[52] Providers can then offer medical advice, being careful not to discount their belief of cause and effect even if it seems scientifically unlikely. Including their understanding of causes as a component of care can be expeditious. Instead of asking "Do you understand?," one can ask the patient to teach back information to gauge whether it was understood.[53]

Table 2
Best practice in working with interpreters

Timing	Key Recommendations
Pre-encounter	Patient[a] preferences • Arrange for an interpreter that aligns with the patient's region/dialect (eg, Sudanese Arabic is not the same as Iraqi Arabic) and gender preferences Prep the interpreter • Brief the interpreter on appointment goals and topics to be covered • Review roles and expectations with interpreter • Remind the interpreter that it is acceptable to take notes during the appointment to ensure accuracy of their interpretation, and that they should feel comfortable asking for clarification or to slow down Practice cultural humility • Ask the interpreter to teach greetings in the patient's language, and review culturally acceptable vs offensive gestures, phrases, etc (eg, shaking hands with opposite gender)
During the encounter	Arrangement of physical space • Be mindful of the interpretation format (in-person, telephonic, video) and arrange participants' seating to optimize patient-provider communication and rapport building, and not exacerbate power differentials Introduction • Introduce the provider (ideally in the patient's language). Introduce anyone else in the room to the patient and confirm it is okay for them to be present • Have the patient and anyone accompanying patient introduce themselves and their relationship • Outline the purpose of the visit and routine to be completed • Allow the interpreter to introduce himself/herself and the interpreter's role • Emphasize this is a conversation whereby patient should intervene whenever they choose Manner of speaking • Speak evenly, concisely, and slowly (no shouting) in first person directly to the patient and family • Pause every 2–3 sentences so the interpreter can interpret • Use appropriate tone. Encourage interpreter to interpret provider's and patient's tone • Talk directly with the patient, not to the interpreter Content • Ensure that all content being said is interpreted (eg, by the patient, family members, medical assistants) • Preface difficult questions with recognition of their difficulty, emphasizing they are asked of everyone • Questions that demand more than simply a yes or no answer are preferable • Think about what to say beforehand to avoid stumbling over words, making contradictory statements, or asking multiple questions at one time • Avoid jargon, ambiguous questions, and oversimplification • Images (eg, Google images) are a powerful mechanism for conveying a great deal of information in a comprehensive way; ask the interpreter to assist with translating information in the images • Do not make assumptions about patients' health and cultural practices Checking in with the patient and patient's family • At regular intervals check with the patient (through assessing body language, asking questions, requesting patient to teach back information,

(continued on next page)

Table 2 (continued)	
Timing	**Key Recommendations**
	and listening) to ensure that the encounter is going well, or if not, to identify and address any issues
	• Ask the patient, not the interpreter, for clarification if the patient's answers are not being understood or if what the patient is describing is unfamiliar
	• If a response to a question seems irrelevant, rephrase the question
	• Before starting a physical examination, describe the process to the patient so that it can be interpreted. See if the patient feels comfortable having an in-person interpreter in the room during the examination or wants them to step out, particularly if no curtain/screen is available
	• *Never* leave the room or finish the appointment without first asking the patient if they have any other questions; if provider is leaving the room, clarify if and when she/he will return
	• Explain all examinations, especially if the interpreter (eg, telephonic) will not be physically present
	Checking in with the interpreter
	• At regular intervals check with the interpreter (through assessing body language, listening, and asking interpreter directly) to ensure that the encounter is going well (eg, that the interpreter is being given enough time to interpret), or if not, to identify and address any issues
	• If interpreter uses English words when interpreting to the patient (eg, "insurance"), ask if there is a corresponding word in the patient's language or confirm that the interpreter has described what the word means
	• Assess whether the interpreter is interpreting all that is being said by paying attention to all conversations (eg, did the patient narrate a long story but the interpreter said to the provider only a few words)
	Respect
	• Provide sufficient time for the interpreter and patients. Concepts in English may not have equivalents in other languages and require more description
	• Do not cut off the interpreter in the middle of their interpretation just because the provider heard the answer they were looking for
	• Listen if interpreter identifies areas of cultural misunderstanding or offense. Ask the interpreter for help rephrasing
	• Avoid uninterpreted side conversations between anyone in the room. This includes between health staff, between family members, and with the interpreter
	• If the child speaks English but the parent does not (or vice versa), allow time for the interpreter to interpret for the parent both the provider's messages and the child's
	• Remain mindful of vicarious traumatization for everyone in the room
	• Remember that the interpreter is not the source of the words. Remain patient even if patient's responses do not make sense, do not answer the question, or are negative
	• Ensure that the interpreter does not advise the patient what to ask or do, and that the patient does not ask the interpreter for advice. This should be decided between provider and patient
	• Talk to the patient as with an English speaker. Do not speak to adults as if they are a child or less intelligent just because they do not speak English
Post-encounter	Debrief with the interpreter and patient
	• Ask the interpreter for feedback about how the appointment went and provide feedback to the interpreter

(continued on next page)

Table 2 (continued)	
Timing	**Key Recommendations**
	• Identify a way for the patient to provide feedback about the interpreter, particularly if they do not want to work with that interpreter again
	Provide language-appropriate materials
	• Provide relevant translated materials, identifying a literate family member if the patient is not literate

[a] Note that where the "patient" is referred to it could also mean the patient's family members, depending on the patient's age.

By checking in with the patient/family during the clinical encounter, providers can enhance communication with families. Some patients may prefer to use a telephonic interpreter or a different interpreter. In addition, interpreters who have worked with the same patients sometimes offer responses to questions that they already "know" the answers to. Although it can be tempting to save time, providers should always ask the patient, not the interpreter, for the patient's medical history.

In addition to checking in directly with the patient, checking in with the interpreter can enhance the quality of communication and may offer learning opportunities for the provider. For instance, if the interpreter seems to be relying on English words to relay information, there may a corresponding word in the patient's language or another word with a similar meaning (a common example is when talking about "health insurance"). Similarly, if the interpreter points out areas of cultural misunderstanding or offense, it is an opportunity to learn how to rephrase the question or statement in an acceptable way.

Effective communication is grounded in respect for the patient and the interpreter. If it seems the interpreter is taking a long time to interpret, keep in mind that concepts in English may not have equivalents in other languages. Moreover, when topics such as trauma are addressed, providers should consider that interpreters may also be immigrants or refugees and/or may have personally experienced or witnessed trauma or torture (see "Vicarious Traumatization"). As a result, the encounter may be difficult for both the interpreter and the patient.

Box 2
Tips for the telephonic interpreter

Telephonic interpreters cannot see nonverbal cues or actions, or what is happening in the room. Be prepared to provide more commentary when working with telephonic interpreters versus in-person/video to ensure they understand the context.

• Introduce the patient and his/her age. This helps the interpreter understand what level of language to use (a 7-year-old is very different from a 16-year-old)

• Have the patient and anyone with the patient introduce themselves and their relationships so that the telephonic interpreter can picture who is in the room

• Describe to the interpreter who is present and their relationship to patient, indicating anyone with good but not fully comprehensive English proficiency

• Narrate what actions are taking place if completing a physical examination or procedure and asking for the patient to follow certain instructions

• Check to ensure the interpreter can hear everyone clearly

Table 3 Physical arrangement of space	
Situation	**Considerations**
Overall	**Be on the patient's level**
	If possible, do not stand towering over the patient; try to sit in a chair that is on the same level as the patient's bed or chair
	Multiple staff
	If multiple health staff members are meeting with the patient, arrange the chairs into a circle so that the patient feels less outnumbered
	Note taking
	If taking notes on computer or written, explain to the patient what will be written down and why, and that it will be kept confidential
	Face the patient
	If using a computer, arrange so provider can view computer as needed while maintaining culturally appropriate eye contact with patient
	If in an examination room, face the patient and make culturally appropriate eye contact. Do not stand with back to the patient, hunched over notes or computer at the counter
In-person interpreter	**Seating arrangements**
	When working with an in-person interpreter, have the interpreter sit to the patient's side or in the best position to be unobtrusive and promote direct communication and eye contact between the provider and the patient[31,51]
Telephonic interpreter	**Move the phone**
	When working with the interpreter by cordless phone, move phone in between the provider and the patient so that both can speak clearly into the phone while still maintaining appropriate eye contact
	Appropriate eye contact
	When using the double "blue phones," ensure that the provider is facing the patient and making appropriate eye contact, not staring off into space over the patient's head or with the body turned away

Post-encounter

At the conclusion of the encounter, feedback offers an opportunity to improve the quality of communication in future encounters. This includes feedback to the interpreter, from the interpreter, and from the patient (particularly if the patient does not want to work with that interpreter again).

Challenges and Ethical Dilemmas

Health care providers who have worked with interpreters may well be familiar with the ethical dilemmas and challenges (**Table 4**). Unfortunately, solutions are complex and heavily depend on each provider's context.[54] Next, some of the most common challenges and some of the solutions that have been successfully implemented are reviewed. Ultimately it is important to keep in mind two points when handling challenges: patients' needs must come first, and everyone in the situation is human.

Vicarious traumatization

Vicarious traumatization represents the emotional repercussions that can occur from hearing others' trauma stories.[55,56] It can occur in interpreters (and providers), who may be especially at risk if they share backgrounds and trauma histories similar to those of the patients. Vicarious traumatization does not happen in a single episode but develops over time. An interpreter may be triggered by the appointment they

Table 4
Challenges and potential solutions for working with interpreters

Challenge/ Ethical Dilemma	Potential Solutions
Vicarious traumatization	Pre-encounter (prepare the interpreter on the topic beforehand) Establish mechanisms for breaks during encounter Check in frequently with patient and interpreter Provide support
Untrained interpreters	Reschedule the appointment with an interpreter Opt for a telephonic interpreter Minimize how much information is discussed until there is a trained interpreter present Review with the untrained individual the rules of interpreting
Gender and ethnicity considerations	Learn about gender and ethnicity dynamics and always ask the patient his or her preference. It is often better to use a telephonic interpreter of the preferred gender and ethnicity than the wrong in-person interpreter
Adolescents	Interview adolescents on their own and check that the adolescent is comfortable to be interviewed with the help of the available interpreter. Explain that confidentiality is certain for the adolescent and only compromised if the adolescent is at risk to self or others
Rare languages	Find out whether video or telephonic interpreters can be accessed. Alert the interpretation company to the need for a certain language. Reach out to local refugee resettlement agencies
Interpreters known within community	Opt for telephonic over in-person interpreters. Have extensive conversations with the interpreter and patients about the interpreter's professional responsibility to maintain confidentiality
Role boundaries	For significant infractions pre-encounter, address them as the appointment is in progress. Address more minor ones during the post-encounter. Notify the interpretation/insurance company of recurring issues
Using children as interpreters	Never use children as interpreters. Reschedule the appointment for a time when an interpreter is available
Patient's refusal of interpreter	Ask questions to ascertain the reasons why the patient is refusing an interpreter. Assess the patient's English abilities. Explain to the patient the importance of an interpreter and that clinic policy dictates that there must be an interpreter. Find out whether a telephonic interpreter is acceptable
Challenges faced by interpreters	Remember that the interpreter is facing issues too. Provide time during and after encounters for the interpreter to let provider know what is going well and what is not going well
Logistical issues	Try to allocate longer appointments for patients needing interpretation. Work with clinical team about who will do what (eg, setting up the interpreter in advance). Cluster appointments for patients from the same family/language when possible

are interpreting. Sometimes the interpreter's reaction may be obvious (eg, she/he starts to cry as the patient relays her story); other times it may be difficult to discern that the interpreter is affected. Interpreters have reported that vicarious traumatization does negatively affect their ability to accurately interpret, making it important for providers to be aware of their interpreters' well-being.[57]

One way to potentially avoid this situation is during the pre-encounter (see **Table 2**). If it appears that the topic could be traumatizing, warn the interpreter ahead of time and check with her or him regarding their comfort level with the topic. This provides the interpreter time to mentally prepare, to think through how the appointment may develop, and to implement coping strategies.[34] Also, during the pre-encounter arrange with the interpreter how to manage if they (or the patient) start to feel over-whelmed—for example, for in-person or video interpreters—and how to signal that they need a break. For telephonic interpreters, it may be possible to call back for a different interpreter.

At times it may be difficult to make these pre-arrangements or the topic may be unan-ticipated. Providers can ask the interpreter to explain to the patient that the interpreter needs to step out of the room for a break. Providers can then check in with the inter-preter after a few moments and offer the choice of continuing or not. If the interpreter opts not to continue, providers can try to find phone interpretation or reschedule the appointment. Following the appointment, providers can take a few moments to debrief with the interpreter about the difficult topics raised—this moment of processing trau-matic stories together may benefit not only the interpreter but also the provider.[34]

Untrained interpreters

As per legal requirements, qualified interpreters are expected for all appoint-ments.[17,58,59] Unfortunately, this is not always the case, sometimes because the fam-ily refuses an interpreter and insists on a family member or friend instead, and other times it is because the meeting is scheduled at the last minute and is urgent, or is ex-pected to be quick or "just one question." Sometimes the patient may speak a rare language and there are no interpreters available. The patient's family members may not speak English either, but may speak a second language that does have an avail-able interpreter. In these instances the interpreter interprets to the family members, who must then interpret what the interpreter says to the patient.

If the urgent need arises to rely on an untrained, ad hoc interpreter, establishing clear rules can facilitate communication (**Box 3**).[60]

Gender and ethnicity considerations

Medical providers can become familiar with gender and ethnicity dynamics and al-ways ask the patient's preference rather than making generalizations.[62] If possible,

---

Box 3
Guidelines for urgently working with untrained interpreters

- Remind the ad hoc interpreter that they must interpret everything the provider says and everything the patient says, exactly as related, in the first person

- Say just 1 or 2 sentences before allowing the person to interpret. Research shows fewer errors when someone is interpreting fewer than 20 words at a time[61]

- Encourage the ad hoc interpreter to ask provider for clarification and to inform the provider and/or patient if it is necessary to speak more slowly

- Keep the conversation minimal and reschedule the appointment with a qualified interpreter

- Check in frequently with the patient to gauge understanding of what is being communicated, not merely asking if she/he understands, but through teach-back questions such as "What are the options for treatment I've just described?" or "How will you take this medication?"[53]

Data from Centre for Culture, Ethnicity & Health. Using teach-back via an interpreter. 2017. Available at: https://www.ceh.org.au/teachbacknews/. Accessed December 17, 2017; and Sinow CS, Corso I, Lorenzo J, et al. Alterations in Spanish language interpretation during pediatric critical care family meetings. Crit Care Med 2017;45(11):1915–21.

providers can alert the insurance or language contracting company (or advise the patient to alert the insurance company) about the gender or ethnicity preference for an upcoming appointment. If the interpreter ends up being the wrong gender or ethnicity, it is often better to use a telephonic interpreter matching the patient's preference than an in-person interpreter of the wrong gender/ethnicity. When meeting with families, it can be difficult to align gender needs for each person in the family (eg, when the male interpreter only speaks with the husband as is culturally correct for the country of origin). In such a scenario it is important to hear from all family members, particularly the mother, directly. This approach may include respectfully coaching the interpreter and family that the mother must answer directly, or rescheduling the appointment (if the meeting is not urgent) and arranging for a female interpreter.

Adolescents
Adolescents should be interviewed independently during the encounter but often are first interviewed with parents present. Providers should advise the parents, patient, and interpreter that routine best practice care recommends the confidential interview of adolescents.[63,64] Providers can check that the adolescent patient is comfortable being interviewed with the help of the available interpreter, changing to telephonic interpreter if needed. It is important to emphasize to the family, patient, and interpreter that confidentiality is only compromised if the adolescent is at risk to self or others. Even if the adolescent patient speaks English, he or she should never interpret for the parents (see "Using Children as Interpreters").[64]

Rare languages
In the case of a rare language, an insurance company and/or interpretation contractor may be able to locate an interpreter. Sometimes rare language interpreters can be found telephonically or through video. By partnering with local refugee resettlement agencies, providers may be able to identify interpreters who have received medical interpretation training (or can receive this training in the future). If no qualified interpreter can be found, providers can establish rules with the family member or friend who will be interpreting (see **Box 3**).

Interpreters known within the community
When interpreters are known within the community, concerns about confidentiality may emerge. In this case, providers should reiterate role boundaries with both the patient and the interpreter[65] and confirm with both the patient and the interpreter that they are comfortable proceeding with the appointment if it becomes known that they know each other. In some cases, providers and patients may choose to explore whether the interpreter can interpret by phone to establish the semblance of physical distance or instead switch to a telephonic interpreter if possible, and if the concern for confidentiality is not alleviated by these measures.

Role boundaries
Role boundaries refers to ensuring that everyone participating in the interpreted encounter is appropriately fulfilling (and is being adequately supported by others to fulfill) their role. For example, interpreters should maintain their roles of communication professionals rather than acting as patients' friends, and interpreters should not offer medical advice instead of the medical provider. The pre-encounter is useful for reminding both interpreters and patients of the boundaries (keeping in mind that qualified interpreters have been trained in role boundaries, whereas patients may be unaware).[66] During the encounter providers can point out behavior that is and is not

appropriate, or, if more appropriate, speak with the interpreter during the post-encounter. If the interpreter continues overstepping boundaries or does something egregious, providers should report this to the insurance company and/or language contracting company. Also, providers can specifically request a different interpreter or opt for a telephonic over an in-person approach. If the patient asks for the interpreter's phone number, providers can help the interpreter by explaining to the patient that it is against the clinic's policy.

Using children as interpreters
Unequivocally, children younger than 18 years should not be used as interpreters, no matter their level of English fluency. The AAP also opposes using children as interpreters.[25,67] The burden of responsibility and potentially life-threatening consequences if something is misunderstood or interpreted incorrectly is too great. In these cases, providers should find a different interpreter by determining whether the patient's insurance offers interpretation, locating a telephonic interpreter, or rescheduling the appointment if possible.

Patients' refusal of interpreters
If a patient refuses an interpreter, providers should explore why the patient does not want to use an interpreter. It can be helpful for providers to ask under what conditions a patient would feel more comfortable using an interpreter (eg, telephonic vs in-person, or reassurance that the interpreter is from a different part of the United States—although depending on the community's size, geographic distance may not be reassuring). Providers can explain the reasons why an interpreter is necessary, the benefits of using a trained medical interpreter, and concerns about the patient's health if she or he does not use one.[68,69] If an interpreter is not used, providers should speak slowly and check in with the patient frequently by asking teach-back questions to ensure understanding. If the family is refusing an interpreter because one of the parents is fluent in English (eg, the father), providers can explain to the family the importance of using an interpreter so that the English-speaking family member can focus on being part of the family and best supporting their child, rather than having to also worry about interpreting. Organizations should also have a protocol in place for when patients refuse interpreters and what must be done in response (eg, the patient must sign a form stating their refusal to use an interpreter).[70] By advising the patient that it is the organization's policy to use interpretation, patients may agree to use interpreters, but it is important to first understand the reasoning behind their refusal.

Interpreters having issues with providers
It is important to keep in mind that challenges faced during an interpreted encounter are not only one-sided. Interpreters face many challenges in working with providers and patients—for example, with patients who overstep boundaries, providers who treat interpreters and the patient disrespectfully and who do not accept an interpreter's feedback about ways to better communicate, or when the provider makes an error with potentially serious health consequences that only the interpreter notices.[35] Providers should learn best practice tips for working with interpreters and be open to feedback from interpreters.

Logistical issues
Using an interpreter can make appointments longer, and interpretation can be expensive. Booking longer appointments or using cluster scheduling to book the whole family for an initial visit may be helpful, particularly for collecting the family history and

other background information that is the same for each family member. In-person interpreters are ideal for these extended appointments. Private grants may support interpretation costs, local refugee resettlement agencies may have trained interpreters for a competitive rate, and state refugee health coordinators may be able to identify resources.

SUMMARY

Training in working through qualified interpreters should be a standard component of orientation programs at medical schools and hospitals.[43] Likewise, best practice tips and clear instructions for accessing telephonic or video remote interpreters should be readily available throughout hospitals and clinics. A few recent pilot studies to train medical residents in working effectively through interpreters demonstrate providers' desire to further develop skills for meeting the needs of their patients with LEP.[21,27,71] Consensus is needed on the specific curricular needs at each stage from medical school through residency and among hospital staff to reduce disparities, including the nature and timing of continuing education. The increasing diversity of patients with LEP, and rapid evolution and change in the medical and interpreting fields, will demand greater opportunities for dialogue between providers and interpreters on improving communication with patients with LEP. Such interdisciplinary collaboration can help avoid ethical dilemmas, contribute to reducing disparities, and ultimately save time and money.

REFERENCES

1. United States Census Bureau. Detailed languages spoken at home and ability to speak English for the population 5 years and over: 2009-2013. Suitland-Silver Hill (MD): United States Census Bureau; 2015.
2. Flores G. The impact of medical interpreter services on the quality of health care: a systematic review. Med Care Res Rev 2005;62(3):255-99.
3. Lindholm M, Hargraves JL, Ferguson WJ, et al. Professional language interpretation and inpatient length of stay and readmission rates. J Gen Intern Med 2012; 27(10):1294-9.
4. Ku L, Flores G. Pay now or pay later: providing interpreter services in health care. Health Aff (Millwood) 2005;24(2):435-44.
5. Flores G, Abreu M, Barone CP, et al. Errors of medical interpretation and their potential clinical consequences: a comparison of professional versus ad hoc versus no interpreters. Ann Emerg Med 2012;60(5):545-53.
6. LaVeist TA, Gaskin D, Richard P. Estimating the economic burden of racial health inequalities in the United States. Int J Health Serv 2011;41(2):231-8.
7. Best practices, investments needed to communicate effectively with LEP patients. ED Manag 2016;28(9):S1-4.
8. Basu G, Costa VP, Jain P. Clinicians' obligations to use qualified medical interpreters when caring for patients with limited English proficiency. AMA J Ethics 2017;19(3):245-52.
9. Goenka PK. Lost in translation: impact of language barriers on children's healthcare. Curr Opin Pediatr 2016;28(5):659-66.
10. Flores G. Families facing language barriers in healthcare: when will policy catch up with the demographics and evidence? J Pediatr 2014;164(6):1261-4.
11. The National CLAS Standards. Available at: https://minorityhealth.hhs.gov/omh/browse.aspx?lvl=2&lvlid=53. Accessed September 15, 2018.

12. Nageswara Rao AA, Warad DM, Weaver AL, et al. Cross-cultural medical care training and education: a National Survey of Pediatric Hematology/Oncology fellows-in-training and fellowship program directors. J Cancer Educ 2018. [Epub ahead of print]. https://doi.org/10.1007/s13187-018-1326-8.
13. Park ER, Betancourt JR, Kim MK, et al. Mixed messages: residents' experiences learning cross-cultural care. Acad Med 2005;80(9):874–80.
14. CHIA, MMIA and NCIHC joint letter of support, September 2005. Available at: https://www.ncihc.org/ethics-and-standards-of-practice. Accessed January 20, 2018.
15. Lee KC, Winickoff JP, Kim MK, et al. Resident physicians' use of professional and nonprofessional interpreters: a national survey. JAMA 2006;296(9):1050–3.
16. Karliner LS, Jacobs EA, Chen AH, et al. Do professional interpreters improve clinical care for patients with limited English proficiency? A systematic review of the literature. Health Serv Res 2007;42(2):727–54.
17. Campanelli RM. Health and Human Services. Office for Civil Rights. Guidance to federal financial assistance recipients regarding Title VI and the prohibition against national origin discrimination affecting limited English proficient persons—summary. 2003; Available at: https://www.hhs.gov/civil-rights/for-providers/laws-regulations-guidance/guidance-federal-financial-assistance-title-vi/index.html. Accessed June 3, 2018.
18. DeCamp LR, Kuo DZ, Flores G, et al. Changes in language services use by US pediatricians. Pediatrics 2013;132(2):e396–406.
19. Thompson DA, Hernandez RG, Cowden JD, et al. Caring for patients with limited English proficiency: are residents prepared to use medical interpreters? Acad Med 2013;88(10):1485–92.
20. Diamond LC, Schenker Y, Curry L, et al. Getting by: underuse of interpreters by resident physicians. J Gen Intern Med 2009;24(2):256–62.
21. Ikram UZ, Essink-Bot ML, Suurmond J. How we developed an effective e-learning module for medical students on using professional interpreters. Med Teach 2015; 37(5):422–7.
22. Macdonald ME, Carnevale FA, Razack S. Understanding what residents want and what residents need: the challenge of cultural training in pediatrics. Med Teach 2007;29(5):444–51.
23. Kripalani S, Bussey-Jones J, Katz MG, et al. A prescription for cultural competence in medical education. J Gen Intern Med 2006;21(10):1116–20.
24. Accreditation Council for Graduate Medical Education (ACGME). Core competencies. Available at: http://med.stanford.edu/gme/housestaff/all-topics/core_competencies.html. Accessed July 10, 2018.
25. Britton CV, American Academy of Pediatrics Committee on Pediatric Workforce. Ensuring culturally effective pediatric care: implications for education and health policy. Pediatrics 2004;114(6):1677–85.
26. American Academy of Pediatrics. Culturally effective care toolkit chapter 5. Interpreter services. 2018. Available at: https://www.aap.org/en-us/professional-resources/practice-transformation/managing-patients/Pages/chapter-5.aspx. Accessed September 22, 2018.
27. Arif S, Cryder B, Mazan J, et al. Using patient case video vignettes to improve students' understanding of cross-cultural communication. Am J Pharm Educ 2017;81(3):56.
28. Ono N, Kiuchi T, Ishikawa H. Development and pilot testing of a novel education method for training medical interpreters. Patient Educ Couns 2013;93(3):604–11.

29. Refugee Health Technical Assistance Center. Available at: https://refugeehealthta.org/access-to-care/language-access/interpreters-vs-translators/. Accessed September 16, 2018.

30. National Association of Judiciary Interpreters & Translators Code of Ethics and Professional Responsibilities. Available at: https://najit.org/wp-content/uploads/2016/09/NAJITCodeofEthicsFINAL.pdf. Accessed June 29, 2018.

31. García-Beyaert SB, Marjory A, Allen K, et al. The community interpreter: an International textbook. Columbia (MA): Culure and Language Press; 2015.

32. California standards for healthcare interpreting. 2017. Available at: http://www.chiaonline.org/CHIA-Standards. Accessed September 18, 2018.

33. California standards for healthcare interpreters. 2002. Available at: http://www.chiaonline.org/CHIA-Standards. Accessed September 18, 2018.

34. Hsieh E. Provider-interpreter collaboration in bilingual health care: competitions of control over interpreter-mediated interactions. Patient Educ Couns 2010; 78(2):154–9.

35. Hsieh E, Kramer EM. Medical interpreters as tools: dangers and challenges in the utilitarian approach to interpreters' roles and functions. Patient Educ Couns 2012; 89(1):158–62.

36. Wu AC, Leventhal JM, Ortiz J, et al. The interpreter as cultural educator of residents: improving communication for Latino parents. Arch Pediatr Adolesc Med 2006;160(11):1145–50.

37. National Council on Interpreting in Health Care. FAQ—translators and interpreters. Available at: https://www.ncihc.org/faq-for-translators-and-interpreters. Accessed May 28, 2018.

38. Jaramillo J, Snyder E, Dunlap JL, et al. The Hispanic Clinic for Pediatric Surgery: a model to improve parent-provider communication for Hispanic pediatric surgery patients. J Pediatr Surg 2016;51(4):670–4.

39. Fernandez A, Perez-Stable EJ. Doctor, habla Espanol? Increasing the supply and quality of language-concordant physicians for Spanish-speaking patients. J Gen Intern Med 2015;30(10):1394–6.

40. Parker MM, Fernandez A, Moffet HH, et al. Association of patient-physician language concordance and glycemic control for limited-English proficiency Latinos with type 2 diabetes. JAMA Intern Med 2017;177(3):380–7.

41. Steinberg EM, Valenzuela-Araujo D, Zickafoose JS, et al. The "battle" of managing language barriers in health care. Clin Pediatr 2016;55(14):1318–27.

42. National standards for culturally and linguistically appropriate services in health and health care: a blueprint for advancing and sustaining CLAS policy and practice. 2013. Available at: https://www.thinkculturalhealth.hhs.gov/clas/blueprint. Accessed December 10, 2018.

43. Huang JJ, Karen C, Regenstein M, et al. Talking with patients: how hospitals use bilingual clinicians and staff to care for patients with language needs (issue brief: survey findings). Washington, DC: Department of Health Policy, School of Public Health and Health Services, The George Washington University; 2009.

44. Diamond LC, Luft HS, Chung S, et al. "Does this doctor speak my language?" Improving the characterization of physician non-English language skills. Health Serv Res 2012;47(1 Pt 2):556–69.

45. Tang G, Lanza O, Rodriguez FM, et al. The Kaiser Permanente Clinician Cultural and Linguistic Assessment Initiative: research and development in patient-provider language concordance. Am J Public Health 2011;101(2):205–8.

46. Language Services Action Kit: interpreter services in health care settings for people with limited English proficiency. 2004. Available at: https://www.commonwealthfund. org/sites/default/files/documents/___media_files_publications_fund_report_2002_ may_providing_language_interpretation_services_in_health_care_settings__exa mples_from_the_field_lep_actionkit_reprint_0204_pdf. Accessed December 10, 2018.

47. Chen AH, Youdelman MK, Brooks J. The legal framework for language access in healthcare settings: Title VI and beyond. J Gen Intern Med 2007;22(Suppl 2): 362–7.

48. Gulf Coast Jewish Family & Community Services' National Partnership for Community Services. Working with interpreters: service provision with torture survivors. Available at: https://gulfcoastjewishfamilyandcommunityservices.org/wp-content/uploads/2018/04/Working-with-Interpreters.pdf. Accessed August 3, 2018.

49. Caring for Kids New to Canada. Using interpreters in health care settings. 2018. Available at: https://www.kidsnewtocanada.ca/care/interpreters. Accessed August 24, 2018.

50. Haffner L. National Council on Interpreting in Health Care working papers series. Guide to interpreter positioning in health care settings. 2003. Available at: https:// www.ncihc.org/resources. Accessed January, 18, 2018.

51. National Council on Interpreting in Health Care. Guide to interpreter positioning in health care settings 2003. Available at: https://www.ncihc.org/publications. Accessed July 25, 2018.

52. Kleinman A, Benson P. Anthropology in the clinic: the problem of cultural competency and how to fix it. PLoS Med 2006;3(10):e294.

53. Centre for Culture, Ethnicity & Health. Using teach-back via an interpreter. 2017. Available at: https://www.ceh.org.au/teachbacknews/. Accessed December 17, 2017.

54. Bancroft M. Community interpreting. A profession rooted in social justice. In: Mikkelson HJ, Jourdenais R, editors. The Routledge handbook of interpreting. New York: Routledge; 2015. p. 217–35.

55. Pearlman LAM, McKay L. Vicarious trauma. 2008. Available at: https://www. headington-institute.org/topic-areas/125/trauma/246/vicarious-trauma. Accessed September 15, 2018.

56. Valero-Garcés C. Emotional and psychological effects on interpreters in public services. a critical factor to bear in mind. Translation Journal 2005;9(3). Available at: http://accurapid.com/journal/33ips.htm. Accessed August 24, 2018.

57. Lai M, Georgina H, Mulayim S. Vicarious trauma among interpreters. International Journal of Interpreter Education 2015;7(1):3–22.

58. President Clinton's Executive Order 13166. August 11, 2000. Improving access to services for persons with limited English proficiency. 2000. Available at: https://www. justice.gov/crt/federal-coordination-and-compliance-section-180. Accessed August 9, 2018.

59. Department of Health and Human Services Office for Civil Rights (OCR). Guidance and standards on language access services for Medicare providers 2010. Available at: http://oig.hhs.gov/oei/reports/oei-05-10-00050.pdf. Accessed September 23, 2018.

60. Gray B, Hilder J, Stubbe M. How to use interpreters in general practice: the development of a New Zealand toolkit. J Prim Health Care 2012;4(1):52–61. A1-8.

61. Sinow CS, Corso I, Lorenzo J, et al. Alterations in Spanish language interpretation during pediatric critical care family meetings. Crit Care Med 2017;45(11): 1915–21.

62. Hadziabdic E, Hjelm K. Working with interpreters: practical advice for use of an interpreter in healthcare. Int J Evid Based Healthc 2013;11(1):69–76.

63. Hirani K, Cherian S, Mutch R, et al. Identification of health risk behaviours among adolescent refugees resettling in Western Australia. Arch Dis Child 2018;103(3): 240–6.

64. Immigrant adolescent health, Part 2: Guidance for clinicians. Caring for Kids New to Canada Available at: https://www.kidsnewtocanada.ca/culture/adolescent-health-guidance-for-clinicians. Accessed December 29, 2018.

65. National Council on Interpreting in Health Care. National standards of practice for interpreters in health care. Washington, DC: NCIHC; 2005.

66. ISSOP Migration Working Group. ISSOP position statement on migrant child health. Child Care Health Dev 2018;44(1):161–70.

67. Hunt DB. Newly adopted anti-discrimination changes to ACA represent biggest changes in the law of language access in nearly twenty years. Available at: https://www.cmelearning.com/new-2016-aca-rules-significantly-affect-the-law-of-language-access/. Accessed December 28, 2018.

68. Moch RN, Hogai G, Tariq Fareed M. Incorporating medical interpretation into your practice. 2014. Available at: https://www.aafp.org/fpm/2014/0300/p16.pdf. Accessed December 29, 2018.

69. Quan K, Jessica L. The high costs of language barriers in medical malpractice. Available at: https://healthlaw.org/resource/the-high-costs-of-language-barriers-in-medical-malpractice/. Accessed December 21, 2018.

70. Newnum G. 4 Best practices to reduce patient refusal of interpreters. CyraCom Language Services Blog: CyraCom. Available at: http://blog.cyracom.com/4-best-practices-to-reduce-patient-refusal-of-interpreters. Accessed January 2, 2019.

71. McEvoy M, Santos MT, Marzan M, et al. Teaching medical students how to use interpreters: a three year experience. Med Educ Online 2009;14:12.

Building a Global Health Workforce in North America

Andrew P. Steenhoff, MBBCh, DCH(UK), FCPaed(SA)[a],*, Stephen Ludwig, MD[b]

KEYWORDS

• Global child health • Local global • Medical education • Pediatric • Competencies

KEY POINTS

• There are many challenges to providing excellent health care both globally and locally.
• To meet these challenges, there needs to be a well-trained, committed workforce in place. That workforce is currently inadequate.
• Pediatricians and pediatric institutions of all sizes need to dedicate themselves to filling this workforce gap.
• Defining the important competencies and finding ways to teach them is critical to making a needed culture change.

INTRODUCTION

The health of children across the world is critical to the continued and improved existence of our world as we know it. Therefore, this outcome is in part the responsibility of all pediatricians and of every department of pediatrics and pediatric governing body.
— *American Board of Pediatrics Global Health Task Force*[1]

Digital technology and modern travel have transformed our world into a global village, tightly connected by an electronic nervous system and the ability to travel almost anywhere within 24 hours.[2,3] Through the impact of the media and the Internet, events in 1 part of the world can be experienced elsewhere in real time, which is what human experience was like when we lived in small villages.[2] One impact of our interconnected global village is enhanced awareness of the needs of children in all settings, which has generated unprecedented interest and action to realize health equity for all children.

Globally, significant progress in health equity for children has been made, but much work remains. In 2017, 5.4 million children less than age 5 died of preventable or treatable conditions.[4] Despite these staggering numbers, the world has made impressive

---

Disclosures: None to declare.
[a] The Children's Hospital of Philadelphia, 3615 Civic Center Boulevard, Suite 1202 ARC, Philadelphia, PA 19104-4318, USA; [b] GME Office, The Children's Hospital of Philadelphia, 3401 Civic Center Boulevard, Philadelphia, PA 19104, USA
* Corresponding author.
E-mail address: steenhoff@email.chop.edu

Pediatr Clin N Am 66 (2019) 687–696
https://doi.org/10.1016/j.pcl.2019.02.013

progress in child survival over the last 30 years: 1 in 26 children died before reaching age 5 in 2017, compared with 1 in 11 in 1990.[4] Similarly, among older children and young adolescents (aged 5–14), mortalities dropped by more than 50% since 1990, although almost 1 million children died in this age group in 2017 alone.[4] Global health (GH), defined "as collaborative transnational research and action for promoting health for all," has emerged as a distinct discipline to address health equity on a global scale.[5]

This article makes the case for building a pediatric GH workforce in North America as well as summarizing current efforts and highlighting deficiencies. The authors advocate for training a workforce of medical providers for global child health (GCH), both for domestic "local global" and for "international global child health" settings. Currently available training resources and approaches for medical students, residents, fellows, pediatricians, and other health practitioners are summarized.

Although the article primarily discusses training pediatricians (given that this is the authors' area of expertise), in building a global workforce, all medical providers who care for children and families are equally important. These providers include family and internal medicine physicians, nurses, and many other health practitioners. Most of the principles and concepts discussed apply to all medical providers, but the authors acknowledge that there likely are excellent models that have not been mentioned. It is hoped this article will stimulate further discussion and facilitate sharing of effective interprofessional GH training models.

Defining the Landscape

In a North American setting, international "global health" involves populations based in low- and middle-income countries. GCH work usually occurs in the context of a GCH partnership, details of which are summarized in a recent literature-based, expert consensus review.[6] Domestic "local global" health involves health of marginalized and underserved populations in a high-income country (HIC), like the United States.[7] **Table 1** summarizes the 7 critical components that 1 group of GH educators consider ideal for a "local global health" program.[7] The fields of "global child health" and domestic "local global" child health share important themes, as summarized in **Fig. 1**, and some experts have argued that international "global health" and domestic "local global" practitioners are one and the same.[8] The authors agree that skills are transferable between these 2 fields, and, for the purposes of this paper, the 2 groups are seen as synonymous.

Need for a Culture Change

A culture change in North American medical and pediatric training institutions is urgently needed; GCH is now a mainstream activity for medical students, pediatric trainees, and pediatricians.[9,10] In 2018, nearly a third of US and Canadian medical students participated in an international GH elective, and in 2015, a quarter of US pediatric residency programs had a GH track with 42% of programs reporting GCH partnerships across 153 countries.[9,11] GCH skills should be included in the core skill set acquired by each pediatric trainee. In decades past, GCH may have been seen as a "hobby for some," a "fringe activity," or the "domain of missionaries, religious groups, development agencies and the Peace Corps." However, in 2019, trainees in medical school, pediatrics, and other health fields clamor for GCH training, and there is a reawakening and enhancement of community engagement by universities and departments of pediatrics. Similarly, many experienced pediatric practitioners from HIC feel a calling to improve the health of all children regardless of the child's geographic location.[10] The mission of North American departments of pediatrics is to improve child health through education, clinical practice, research, and advocacy.[12] This mission is also broadening to include improving health for all children as departments

Table 1
The 7 critical components that 1 group of global health educators consider ideal for a domestic "local global health" program

Element	Explanation
Community engagement	Local global programs should be more than a teaching tool; they should meet a need in the community. This requires engaging the local community in the process, a central tenet of community engagement and GH. Community engagement ensures that new initiatives have value for both communities and students
Global frameworks/local solutions and transferable skills	Students should be taught universally recognized health frameworks, such as the social determinants of health, international human rights law, ethics (clinical, research, professional), cultural competence, program development, and program evaluation with a practical focus on how to adapt these frameworks to the needs of a particular community. These skills should be taught along with (or as part of) professional skills to form a set of transferable skills that can be adapted to vulnerable populations wherever they exist
Focus on social justice and health care disparities	The availability of adequate health care is almost always affected by socioeconomic factors; hence, local global programs must maintain a focus on health disparities and social justice
Bidirectional learning	Understanding health and health care in context is crucial to reciprocal sharing of successful local strategies in a way that has not occurred historically, and thus, local global programs should teach students the value of bidirectional learning and how to adapt tested strategies to meet local needs
Experiential/clinical learning	Local global programs should offer students the opportunity to step out of the classroom and develop their ability to work with individuals, groups, and organizations that are new to them. A local global program can provide this opportunity. For graduate students, this can take the form of clinical work in which students practice their professional skills under appropriate supervision. Experiential learning can also expose students to community engagement through structured observation, interaction, and service
Interprofessional approach	Improving health requires a broad array of multidisciplinary and multifaceted methods. Local global programs should teach students the value of an interprofessional approach by incorporating faculty and students from different schools in a single program
Reflective component	There is value in structured reflective opportunities for students taking part in immersion experiences. Reflection is critical to guide the learning process and facilitate personal growth

Data from Rowthorn V. Global/local: what does it mean for global health educators and how do we do it? Ann Glob Health 2015;81(5):593–601.

respond to growing calls, both domestic and international, for health equity.[1,12–14] In sum, GCH is now within the purview of every pediatrician in North America.

Global Health Competencies in Medical Education

In order to train a GH workforce, core GH competencies need to be defined, for GH learners of all levels. Over the last 12 years, several groups have defined and discussed GH competencies for different learners.[15–26] Developing consensus on GH

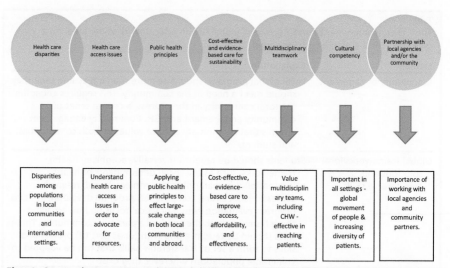

Fig. 1. Seven themes connecting "global" and domestic "local global" health. CHW, community health workers. (*Data from* Evert J, DP, Hall T. Developing global health programming: a guidebook for medical and professional schools. 2nd edition. San Francisco 2014.)

competencies ensures that GH students at different training institutions are exposed to similar basic levels of training.[15]

Defining competencies in GH has been an active area of research. For medical students, in 2007, 3 domains of GH competency were proposed by the American Society of Tropical Medicine and Hygiene Committee on Medical Education: global burden of disease, traveler's medicine, and immigrant health.[16] A 2011 review highlighted the imperative to document GH educational competencies and approaches used in medical schools and the need to facilitate greater consensus among medical educators on appropriate GH training for future physicians.[15] Of 15 GH competencies mentioned in the review, the most commonly discussed ones included an understanding of the global burden of disease; travel medicine; health care disparities between countries; immigrant health; primary care within diverse cultural settings; and skills to better interface with different populations, cultures, and health care systems.[15]

In 2013, recognizing the rapid expansion of GH programs and the lack of standardized competencies and curricula to guide these programs, the Consortium of Universities for Global Health (CUGH) appointed a Global Health Competency Subcommittee charged with identifying broad GH core competencies applicable across disciplines.[17] The CUGH subcommittee wisely recognized a need to distinguish between levels of GH competency to reflect differences in the educational and professional goals of trainees: 4 GH competency levels were proposed (**Fig. 2**), from global citizen level (most basic) to the advanced level. These competency levels are applicable across disciplines and professional categories.

The final list of individual GH competencies varied by level with more competencies in the higher levels. For example, the 8 domains for global citizen were global burden of disease; globalization of health and health care; social and environmental determinants of health; collaboration, partnering, and communication; ethics; professional practice; health equity and social justice; and sociocultural and political awareness.[17] For the program-oriented basic operational level, in addition to the 8 domains for

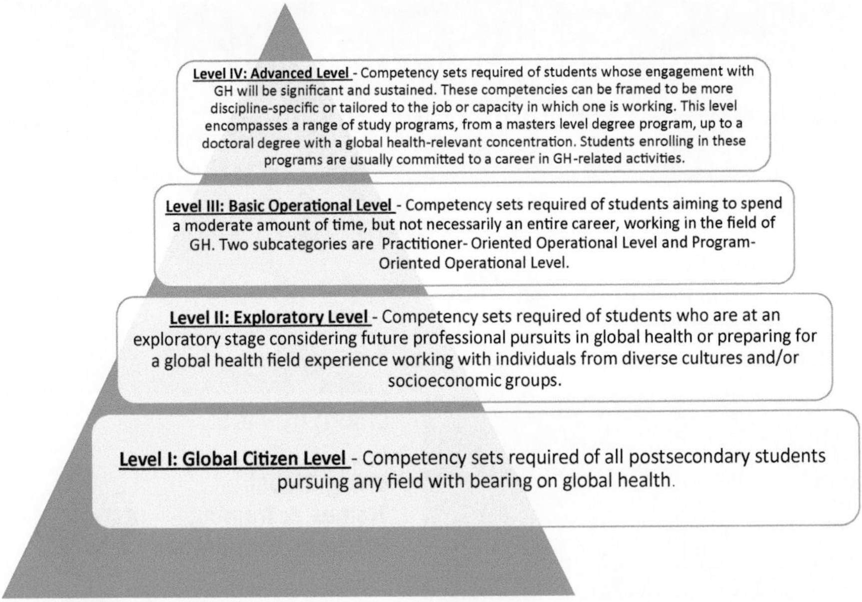

Fig. 2. Levels of GH competency: the 4 levels proposed by the CUGH. (*Data from* Jogerst K, Callender B, Adams V, et al. Identifying interprofessional global health competencies for 21st-century health professionals. Ann Glob Health 2015;81(2):239–47.)

global citizen level, 3 additional domains were included (giving a total of 11 competency domains): capacity strengthening, program management, and strategic analysis.

A recent review of GH competencies for postgraduate public health education also described 11 GH competency domains; these competency domains primarily referred to 3 main aspects: one focused on burden of disease and determinants of health; a second focused on core public health skills, including policy development, analysis, and program management; and a third, that could be classified as "soft skills" and included collaboration, partnering, communication, professionalism, capacity building, and political awareness.[18]

Subsequently, in 2017, the CUGH Inter-professional Global Health Competencies were used to develop a GH milestones tool based on the 11 GH domains; this tool will next be tested for validity and utility.[19] Although it is encouraging seeing the development of medical education scholarship in the field of GH, some experts have called for improved methods of curriculum evaluation and enhanced publication guidelines to positively impact the quality of research in this area.[20]

Global Health in Pediatric Education: an Implementation Guide for Pediatric Program Directors

Recognizing GH as an emerging area of priority in pediatrics, the American Board of Pediatrics recently convened a group of pediatric GH experts to develop GH resources to support educators and pediatricians. The group created "Global health in pediatric education: an implementation guide for pediatric program directors." This outstanding guide, which is free to download, is a comprehensive, practical resource for incorporating GH education into pediatric residency and fellowship programs.[27] **Fig. 3** summarizes the contents. Although specifically developed for

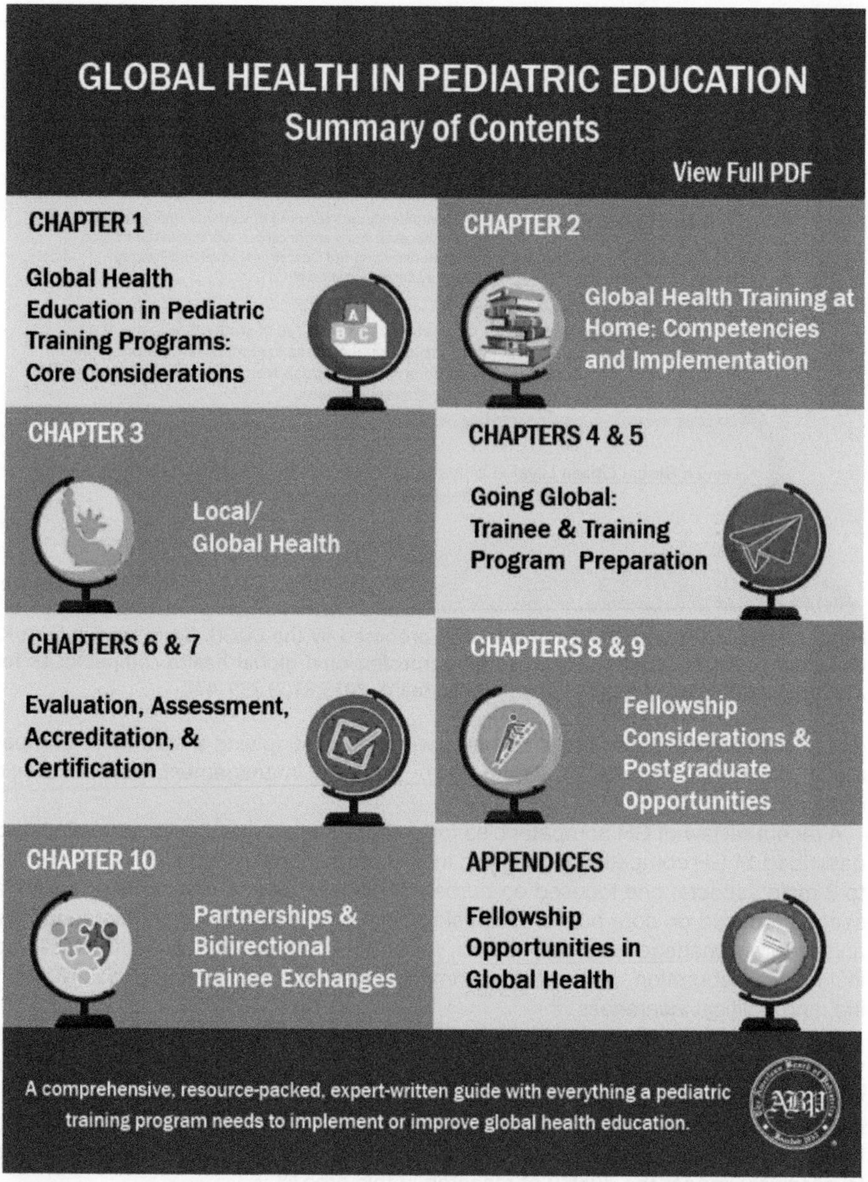

Fig. 3. Infographic of the "Global health in pediatric education: an implementation guide for pediatric program directors." (*Data from* St Clair N, Abdul-Mumin A, Banker S, et al. Global health in pediatric education: an implementation guide for program directors. American Board of Pediatrics Global Health Task Force Publication, in collaboration with the American Academy of Pediatrics Section on International Child Health and the Association of Pediatric Program Directors Global Health Learning Community. September 2018. Available at: http://www.abp.org/ghpdguidehome, Accessed February 17, 2019.)

pediatric residency and fellowship program directors, many of the principles are applicable to other GH learners.

Centers of Global and Urban Health

As the discipline of GH has developed over the last 20 years, so too GH centers have mushroomed at universities, at medical schools, and in some children's hospitals. Similarly, many pediatric institutions now have centers dedicated to local global populations, including centers for the urban child and immigrant and refugee clinics. These centers demonstrate institutional commitment to the underserved, help create a GH career path for GH-focused faculty, and represent an excellent learning environment for GH learners.

How Do We Build a Global Health Workforce?

To meet the needs of global and local child health, there needs to be a well-trained, committed workforce in place. That workforce is currently inadequate. Medical and other health schools, pediatric institutions of all sizes, and pediatricians need to dedicate themselves to filling this workforce gap. With a focus on meeting the needs of children and families, training this workforce entails activities in all of these groups: medical students, residents (at least pediatrics, family medicine, internal medicine), fellows, other health practitioners, and upskilling current practitioners (eg, experienced pediatricians or near retirement professionals who wish to contribute their skills to the GH workforce).

The most common educational approaches for teaching GH are didactics and experiential learning. GH topics should be integrated within medical school curricula. Scholars have called for "more detailed documentation of global health educational approaches if the literature is to serve as a resource for medical schools developing new programs."[15] There is a vast array of options for training in GH; many of these can be accessed by learners from undergraduate to experienced faculty. Training opportunities in GH include university, medical school, or pediatric GH centers, urban experiences, including refugee and immigrant clinics, rotations at city health departments, including tuberculosis clinics, mentorship, summer research experiences, the Indian Health Service, training in language services, and cross-cultural competencies. There are many innovative GH programs that seek to help address the health needs of underserved communities and discussion with a local experienced GH mentor can often yield a treasure trove of opportunities; an example is Alaska's medical school, which is a collaborative medical school between universities in 5 northwestern states – Washington, Wyoming, Alaska, Montana, and Idaho, called the WWAMI collaborative, which is known for delivering high-quality primary care.[28]

There are also resident and fellow-specific GH training opportunities. For residents, GH tracks provide an opportunity to have a mentored, concentrated GH learning experience in the international, local, or both settings. Similarly, for fellows, there are dedicated pediatric GH fellowships as well as GH tracks in subspecialty fellowships.[27] Depending on funding models and the curriculum, current pediatric GH fellowships vary from 2- to 3-year immersive international GH experiences to 1- to 2-year intermittent 4- to 6-month GH experiences punctuated by time in the United States.[29,30] Pediatric GH fellowships focus on acquiring skills in different domains, including research, clinical care, teaching, and advocacy. Although the current pediatric GH fellowship landscape and approach are highly flexible and foster innovation, there may be a role in the future for setting core competencies for pediatric GH fellowships. In family medicine, for example, a panel of GH experts has developed a mission statement and identified 6 domains for family medicine GH fellowships: patient care, medical knowledge, professionalism, communication and leadership, teaching, and scholarship; each domain includes a set of core and program-specific competencies.[23]

Although many programs have been established to afford US physicians opportunities to travel abroad, few have established reciprocal travel for international colleagues to come to the United States. More bidirectional opportunities will help to expand the workforce always with the caveat that training opportunities should not detract from trainees taking their newly gained experiences back to their home countries. Similarly, there is a role for North American national medical education organizations to consider how to facilitate building a GH workforce in North America while also participating in harmonizing and improving training standards internationally. An example of the latter is the Accreditation Council for Graduate Medical Education (ACGME) and its affiliate group ACGME-International (ACGME-I), who accredit international graduate medical education programs and seek to "advance health care by assessing the quality of physicians' education through a voluntary, peer-review evaluation process that benefits the public and improves the quality of teaching, learning, research, and professional practice throughout the world."[31]

Pediatric practitioners have a range of opportunities to participate in GCH, clearly summarized in a recent review.[10] In most situations, there is also opportunity for less GH-experienced pediatricians to learn from more seasoned GH practitioners. In addition, many volunteer organizations like the Peace Corps accept older applicants, provide GH training, and afford volunteers a wonderful range of GH opportunities.[32]

Current Deficiencies in Building a Global Health Workforce in North America

Although significant progress is being made in GCH, there are many opportunities to accelerate progress for the benefit of children. Defining the important GH competencies and finding ways to teach them are critical to making a needed culture change. In addition, improvements in the scientific rigor are needed in assessing the educational impact of GH on trainees, including improved methods of curriculum evaluation and creating an environment of continuous evidence-based quality improvement. Similarly, greater development of GH-expert faculty must be ensured through high-quality GH training and mentorship, particularly of residents and fellows. Clear career tracks are also needed for GH educators, clinicians, and researchers. The important role that international medical graduates (IMGs) play caring for the underserved in the United States is often underappreciated, 25% of US pediatricians and 27% of US pediatric subspecialists are IMGs. IMGs frequently practice in rural and underserved areas, caring for marginalized communities. The unintended negative impact of national policies, such as the recent travel ban that affected people from certain countries, adversely impacted many medical trainees and some in the GH workforce.

SUMMARY

GCH is now within the purview of every pediatrician in North America. There are many challenges to providing excellent health care both globally and locally. To meet these challenges, there needs to be a well-trained, committed workforce in place. That workforce is currently inadequate. Pediatricians and pediatric institutions of all sizes need to dedicate themselves to filling this workforce gap. Defining the important competencies and finding ways to teach them are critical to making a needed culture change.

REFERENCES

1. Butteris SM, Haig V. Mind the gap: lessons from one board's focus on global health. Available at: https://static1.squarespace.com/static/5581c84de4b08614acb89b1f/t/59cd37c52278e76a7ff30a5e/1506621385211/09.26_0915_Butteris_Haig_MOC-LLSA-032.pdf. Accessed February 21, 2019.
2. Marshall McLuhan predicts the global village. Available at: https://livinginternet.com/i/ii_mcluhan.htm. Accessed February 16, 2019.
3. UNICEF: The state of the world's children in 2017 - children in a digital world. Available at: https://www.unicef.org/sowc2017/. Accessed February 17, 2019.
4. UNICEF: Under five mortality 2017. Available at: https://data.unicef.org/topic/child-survival/under-five-mortality/. Accessed February 17, 2019.
5. Beaglehole R, Bonita R. What is global health? Glob Health Action 2010;3:5142.
6. Steenhoff AP, Crouse HL, Lukolyo H, et al. Partnerships for Global Child Health. Pediatrics 2017;140(4).
7. Rowthorn V. Global/local: what does it mean for global health educators and how do we do it? Ann Glob Health 2015;81(5):593–601.
8. Evert J, Drain P, Hall T. Developing global health programming: a guidebook for medical and professional schools. 2nd edition. San Francisco (CA): Global Health Collaborations Press; 2014.
9. Butteris SM, Schubert CJ, Batra M, et al. Global health education in US pediatric residency programs. Pediatrics 2015;136(3):458–65.
10. Arora G, Esmaili E, Pitt MB, et al. Pediatricians and global health: opportunities and considerations for meaningful engagement. Pediatrics 2018;142(2).
11. Association of American Medical Colleges medical school graduation questionnaire: 2018 all schools summary report. Available at: https://www.aamc.org/download/490454/data/2018gqallschoolssummaryreport.pdf. Accessed February 18, 2019.
12. Gladding SP, McGann PT, Summer A, et al, Global Health Task Force of the American Board of Pediatrics. The collaborative role of north american departments of pediatrics in global child health. Pediatrics 2018;142(1) [pii:e20172966].
13. Sachs JD. From millennium development goals to sustainable development goals. Lancet 2012;379(9832):2206–11.
14. AAP agenda for children: health equity. Available at: https://www.aap.org/en-us/about-the-aap/aap-facts/AAP-Agenda-for-Children-Strategic-Plan/Pages/AAP-Agenda-for-Children-Strategic-Plan-Health-Equity.aspx. Accessed February 17, 2019.
15. Battat R, Seidman G, Chadi N, et al. Global health competencies and approaches in medical education: a literature review. BMC Med Educ 2010;10:94.
16. Houpt ER, Pearson RD, Hall TL. Three domains of competency in global health education: recommendations for all medical students. Acad Med 2007;82(3):222–5.
17. Jogerst K, Callender B, Adams V, et al. Identifying interprofessional global health competencies for 21st-century health professionals. Ann Glob Health 2015;81(2):239–47.
18. Sawleshwarkar S, Negin J. A review of global health competencies for postgraduate public health education. Front Public Health 2017;5:46.
19. Douglass KA, Jacquet GA, Hayward AS, et al. Development of a global health milestones tool for learners in emergency medicine: a pilot project. AEM Educ Train 2017;1(4):269–79.

20. Bills CB, Ahn J. Global health and graduate medical education: a systematic review of the literature. J Grad Med Educ 2016;8(5):685–91.
21. Arthur MA, Battat R, Brewer TF. Teaching the basics: core competencies in global health. Infect Dis Clin North Am 2011;25(2):347–58.
22. Cherniak W, Latham E, Astle B, et al. Visiting trainees in global settings: host and partner perspectives on desirable competencies. Ann Glob Health 2017;83(2): 359–68.
23. Rayess FE, Filip A, Doubeni A, et al. Family medicine global health fellowship competencies: a modified delphi study. Fam Med 2017;49(2):106–13.
24. Wilson L, Harper DC, Tami-Maury I, et al. Global health competencies for nurses in the Americas. J Prof Nurs 2012;28(4):213–22.
25. Warren N, Breman R, Budhathoki C, et al. Perspectives of nursing faculty in Africa on global health nursing competencies. Nurs Outlook 2016;64(2):179–85.
26. Nordhues HC, Bashir MU, Merry SP, et al. Graduate medical education competencies for international health electives: a qualitative study. Med Teach 2017; 39(11):1128–37.
27. St Clair N, Abdul-Mumin A, Banker S, et al. Global health in pediatric education: an implementation guide for program directors. Chapel Hill (NC): American Board of Pediatrics Global Health Task Force Publication, in collaboration with the American Academy of Pediatrics Section on International Child Health and the Association of Pediatric Program Directors Global Health Learning Community. September 2018. Available at: http://www.abp.org/ghpdguidehome, Accessed February 17, 2019.
28. Alaska WWAMI program. Available at: https://www.uaa.alaska.edu/academics/ college-of-health/departments/wwami/. Accessed February 19, 2019.
29. David N. Pincus global health fellowship. Available at: https://www.chop.edu/ pediatric-fellowships/global-health-center/fellowship. Accessed February 19, 2019.
30. UMASS pediatric global health fellowship. Available at: https://www.umassmed. edu/pediatrics/pediatrics-global-health-fellowship/. Accessed February 19, 2019.
31. ACGME International Homepage. Available at: https://www.acgme-i.org/. Accessed February 21, 2019.
32. Peace corps - volunteering at 50 plus. Available at: https://www.peacecorps.gov/ volunteer/is-peace-corps-right-for-me/50plus/. Accessed February 19, 2019.